Every Body Can Learn

Every Body Can Learn

Engaging the
Bodily-Kinesthetic
Intelligence in
the Everyday Classroom

Marilyn Nikimaa Patterson

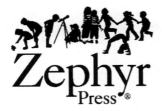

Zephyr
Press®

REACHING THEIR HIGHEST POTENTIAL
TUCSON, ARIZONA

Every Body Can Learn
Engaging the Bodily-Kinesthetic Intelligence in the Everyday Classroom

Grades 5–12

©1997 by Marilyn Nikimaa Patterson
Printed in the United States of America

ISBN 1-56976-057-8

Editors: Sonya Manes and Stacey Shropshire
Cover design: Stirling Crebbs
Design and production: Daniel Miedaner
Typesetting: Daniel Miedaner

Zephyr Press
P.O. Box 66006
Tucson, AZ 85728-6006

All rights reserved. No form of this work may be reproduced, transmitted, or recorded without written permission from the publisher.

Library of Congress Cataloging-in-Publication Data
Patterson, Marilyn Nikimaa, 1939-
    Every body can learn : engaging the bodily-kinesthetic
intelligence in the everyday classroom / Marilyn Nikimaa Patterson.
        p. cm.
    Includes bibliographical references.
    ISBN 1-56976-057-8
    1. Activity programs in education. 2. Teaching. 3. Kinesiology.
 4. Mind and body. 5. Learning, Psychology of.   I. Title.
LB1027.25.P38 1996
371.3'9—dc20   96-30261.

*To George Leonard,
a master teacher
of the capacities
of body and mind.*

Acknowledgments

I am especially indebted to the individuals who have allowed me to include adaptations of their work: George Leonard, Jean Houston, and Richard Shope.

I would like to thank my colleagues, Anne Bruetsch, Jaelline Jaffe, and Louise Sample, as well as my husband, Robert D. Patterson, for their unfailing encouragement. A special thank you goes to my students from the past three decades for their curiosity, humor, imagination, and enthusiasm for kinesthetic learning activities.

Illustration Credits

- 2.1: Robert A. Smith, 4408 Moscato Way, Bakersfield, CA 93306. 2.2: National Association for the Deaf, 814 Thayer Ave., Silver Spring, MD 20910.
- 3.1: Robert A. Smith. 3.2, 3.3: *History Alive!* ©1996 Teachers' Curriculum Institute, 2465 Latham Street, Ste. 100, Mountain View, CA 94040, 800 497-6138. 3.4, 3.5, 3.6, 3.7: Interact, 1825 Gillespie Way 100, El Cajon 92020.
- 4.1, 4.2: NASA/Jet Propulsion Laboratory, Pluto Express Educational Outreach, 4800 Oak Grove Drive, Pasadena, CA 91109. (4.1 Adapted by Robert A. Smith.)
- 5.1: George Leonard, *Leonard Energy Training, A Trainer's Manual.* 1983. Energy Training Institute, P. O. Box 258, Mill Valley, CA, 94942. 5.2, 5.3, 5.4: *Brain Gym.* Paul Dennison, Ph.D., P. O. Box 3396, Ventura CA 93001-3303. 5.5, 5.6, 5.7, 5.8: George Leonard, *Leonard Energy Training, A Trainer's Manual.* 1983. Energy Training Institute, P. O. Box 258, Mill Valley, CA, 94942.

Contents

Introduction	1
1. Getting Started	9
2. English and Other Languages	25
3. Social Sciences	43
4. Mathematics and the Natural Sciences	69
5. Study Skills, Self-Management, and Conflict Resolution	91
Appendix: Cross-Referenced Chart of Activities	123
Bibliography	127
Organizations, Publishers, and Presenters	134

Introduction

Great ideas originate in the muscles.
—Thomas Edison

What Is the Bodily-Kinesthetic Intelligence?

Our idea of intelligence has changed dramatically in the last ten years. We used to think that each person was born with a certain level of intelligence that stayed the same throughout life. We thought we could measure this intelligence accurately with standardized tests and express it with a number we called *IQ*. The research of people such as Howard Gardner of Harvard University has changed all that.

We now know that we have several intelligences and that we can help them grow stronger. Gardner has identified seven major intelligences, each of which can keep developing throughout life. You can read the fascinating story of how he came to this insight in his books *Frames of Mind* and *Multiple Intelligences,* so I won't go into detail about it here.

Gardner (1993) defines an intelligence as "the ability to solve problems or fashion products that are of consequence in a particular cultural setting or community" (7). Following is a brief summary of the seven intelligences.

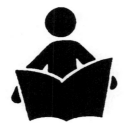

1. The *verbal-linguistic* intelligence involves the use of words. Outstanding writers, orators, and storytellers show a high level of this intelligence, but everyone else has it, too.

Introduction

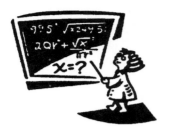

2. The *mathematical-logical* intelligence involves systems of numbers and logic. Scientists, mathematicians, accountants, and computer programmers use this intelligence heavily. However, everyone, even a math-hater, has this intelligence and can develop it.

3. The *visual-spatial* intelligence involves visual images and understanding of three-dimensional space. Mechanical designers, architects, artists, and airline pilots depend on this kind of intelligence. Everyone else uses it every day, too. A blind person uses the spatial component to move from one place to another.

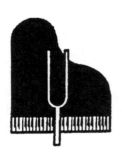

4. The *musical-rhythmic* intelligence encompasses melody, rhythm, and pitch. Clearly, musicians possess a high degree of this intelligence, but speakers of the principal Chinese languages rely on it also, as these languages are tonal. To understand them, a listener has to distinguish among four to ten different spoken tones. If you think you don't have this intelligence because you can't carry a tune, you're wrong. Your musical intelligence shows up even in the rhythm of your step as you walk down the street.

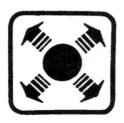

5. The *interpersonal* intelligence allows us to work effectively with other people. Psychologists, personnel managers, parents of large families, and effective business executives frequently exhibit a high degree of this intelligence. Cooperative learning groups often help students refine it.

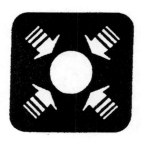

6. The *intrapersonal* intelligence gives us access to the workings of our own minds and emotions. We see intrapersonal intelligence at work in people who demonstrate self-understanding, who set and accomplish goals, and who modify their own moods without depending on external chemicals. If all our young people were strong in this area, they might not have so many drug abuse problems.

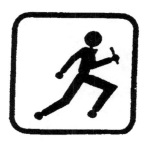

7. The *bodily-kinesthetic* intelligence allows us to solve problems or create worthwhile products using the body or parts of it, such as the hands. An integral aspect of this intelligence is the kinesthetic ("movement-sensing") capacity, the richness of perception built into our neuromuscular system that underlies a great deal of learning, not only that done through physical activities. I discuss this perceptive aspect in detail after I clear up a few common misconceptions about the use of the bodily-kinesthetic intelligence.

Many of us tend to associate the bodily-kinesthetic intelligence with athletic superstars, mechanics, or craftspeople. We often assume that it belongs exclusively to the never-never land of TV sports, or perhaps in physical education or vocational classes. Or we may think that classrooms need to include bodily-kinesthetic activities only in the early grades. Few of us realize the immense value of these activities in upper grades and in the everyday life of adolescents. Students in middle and high school are going through drastic and bewildering physical changes, and they benefit from any activity that helps them see their bodies as allies. Moreover, the body is a largely neglected ally of the teacher. George Leonard often notes in his seminars: "The body

Introduction

is the ultimate learning device. It has billions of circuits, immediate feedback, and *every student comes equipped with one*" (emphasis mine).

Increasing numbers of scientists are finding that there isn't a clear division between the body and the mind. The mind plays a major role in the health of the body, and the body, in turn, helps determine how effectively the mind works. Many scientists are now beginning to think in terms of the "bodymind," a unity that many traditional cultures have never lost. Serving as a bridge between body and mind, the kinesthetic aspect of the bodily-kinesthetic intelligence lets us receive and interpret the millions of signals, both internal and external, that keep us alive. It's far more than a mere survival mechanism, though. Contemporary research shows us that this intelligence helps us enhance our physical and intellectual functioning in ways we've never thought possible.

In this book are ideas for using the bodily-kinesthetic intelligence to help your students learn English, history, biology, or geometry, as well as other upper-grade subjects.

Why Include Bodily-Kinesthetic Activities in the Academic Classroom?

They benefit students who learn best with the bodily-kinesthetic intelligence. Think of several "problem learners" you've observed. How many of them have trouble sitting still? How many need to touch something to understand it, or learn best from field trips or real-life applications of the subject matter? These students' primary intelligence is probably bodily-kinesthetic. Most classrooms have a good number of these students, but the majority of traditional classroom activities are oriented only to the verbal or analytical intelligence. Kinesthetically oriented kids deserve a reasonable proportion of teaching geared toward their preferred intelligence. Including kinesthetic activities can give those students a two-way information highway that's often missing in traditional classroom practice. Moreover, you can assess these students more accurately through assignments that engage the bodily-kinesthetic intelligence.

They benefit all students. Bodily-kinesthetic activities serve many functions:

- They resemble activities students would do themselves if not in school. These activities offer more sensory input, which holds student attention. Because of this quality, students tend to retain the learning, a benefit even to those whose strength is in another intelligence.

- They often engage other intelligences, as well, especially the interpersonal, the rhythmic element of musical-rhythmic, and the spatial component of visual-spatial intelligences. Such activities promote the integration and enhancement of various intelligences and can improve all areas of sensory perception. If you encourage students to be aware of this process, they discover more about their preferred intelligences. This metaknowledge, in turn, allows students to direct more effectively their stronger intelligences to enhance their less-developed ones.

- Many of them produce long-term rather than short-term recall. You may remember, for example, something you learned in a school play in the third grade, whereas you've forgotten much of the other subject matter of that period. This may be because participation in the play fully activated your kinesthetic sensory system. You probably still remember how to perform certain physical activities, such as riding a bicycle or swimming, even if you haven't practiced for years. Kinesthetic activities in school often produce the same results.

- They seem to activate the right hemisphere of the brain. The right hemisphere tends to perceive things in their totality rather than as individual components and is relatively free of the "editor" that operates on the left side. Using kinesthetic activities along with traditional left-brain classroom strategies helps students see a more complete picture of the subject matter, free themselves from learning inhibitions, and activate a wider range of neural patterns. Some kinesthetic activities help integrate the two

hemispheres, allowing the entire cerebrum to work as a unit, rather than half at a time.
- They help students develop study skills, self-management, and conflict resolution skills. These activities provide experience rather than just precept. Chapter 5 provides more details in this area.

The Purpose of This Book

This book suggests several ways of using kinesthetic activities to make teaching easier and more effective. To implement these activities, you don't have to be a physical education teacher. You don't even have to be strong in this intelligence yourself. You can include a reasonable number of these activities on a regular basis *without* a major restructuring of your teaching approach. Of course, the more you include each of the multiple intelligences, the more thoroughly your students learn, but it's okay to start small.

Each chapter includes descriptions of activities you can put to immediate use in specific subject areas. Areas include English and other languages; social sciences; mathematics and natural sciences; and study skills, self-management, and conflict resolution. I do not include the visual and performing arts, because there are already some fine books available that focus on these areas, notably Gail Herman and Patricia Hollingsworth's *Kinetic Kaleidoscope* and Teresa Benzwie's *A Moving Experience*. I have included optional and sample scripts throughout the book, within certain activities and in the form of subject-specific journeys achieved through the kinesthetic imagination. These scripts are intended as vivid illustrations of new techniques and as examples of structuring devices and discourse. You may choose to follow them faithfully or use them merely as springboards to activities conducted in your own imaginative style. The portions to be spoken to students appear in italic type, and the instructions to you appear in roman type. An ellipsis signifies a pause in which students are given a chance to think or respond.

You can use some of the activities described in this book in more than one subject. For that reason, I include a cross-referenced chart of activities at the end of the book, which suggests the range of subjects appropriate for each activity. If you're a math teacher, for example, you can concentrate on the activities in chapter 4 and also consult the chart to find the other activities that could be applicable to math classes. At the end of the book is a bibliography that includes organizations, publishers, and presenters who are doing outstanding work in these areas.

1 Getting Started

The longest journey begins with the first step.
—Chinese proverb

You don't have to be an expert to make a good beginning. Here are a few suggestions to help you start.

Be Aware of Your Preferred Modes of Learning and Teaching

Do you prefer to learn by seeing, hearing, or doing? Do you like to analyze or to think in metaphors? Do you learn best in a group or alone? Which intelligences do you favor? Are your lesson plans linear and closely organized or spiral and flexible? Keep in mind that there are many different valid modes of teaching. How does your teaching style harmonize with the learning styles of your students?

In schools of education, many of us were taught to stand at the front of the room and expect all students to pay conscientious attention to our words. The teacher and the textbook were considered the prime sources of information. Recent research indicates that sometimes it's more effective for teachers to have students work cooperatively in small groups, processing information from a number of sources. For a time the teacher becomes the "Guide on the Side" rather than the "Sage on the Stage." Several of the activities in this book enable you to assume the guide role while maintaining effective but flexible structure.

Chapter 1

Start with Familiar, Easy Activities

Engaging the bodily-kinesthetic intelligence is much easier than it may seem at first. You may have been using some bodily-kinesthetic activities for years, such as field trips, hands-on projects, skits, and creative book reports. In this book are some of your old standbys, but there is also a wealth of new ideas you can introduce easily into the classroom. Although you may think that using these activities will complicate your job, they will actually facilitate it.

Many teachers quail at the idea of using physical activities in an academic classroom. They may imagine a classroom in pandemonium, with thirty or more adolescents stumbling over desks or slamming into walls. Nothing could be further from the truth! For students not accustomed to using movement for learning, you can start small, with hands-on activities or with movement limited to a small area. There's even a form of "muscular imagination" students can use that requires little or no physical movement.

Kinesthetic techniques vary widely. This book describes techniques that use the whole body, as well as activities that feature the large muscles, hands-on involvement, kinesthetic imagination, and perception enhancement. The following section gives examples of the various types of activities. In later chapters are detailed descriptions of these and many other activities, categorized by subject. The authors and organizations mentioned are included in the bibliography. A cross-referenced chart (pages 123–25) lists each activity alphabetically, indicating its movement category and the subject areas in which it can be used.

Types of Activities in This Book
Whole-Body

If you're willing to use whole-body activities, there are several that work well in academic classes. A prime example is total physical response (TPR) described in chapter 2. This well-structured, highly effective approach is often used for teaching languages and ESL. Berty Segal and James J. Asher have produced splendid books of lesson plans for using TPR (see the "English and Other Languages" section of the bibliography). Other whole-body techniques include skits and charades.

Large Muscle

A friend of mine teaches Urdu (the national language of Pakistan, which is written in Arabic script) at a university. She has enabled her students to overcome their difficulties in mastering the Arabic alphabet by having them write the letters and words on the chalkboard with the whole arm rather than just the hand. In his *Brain Gym* materials, Paul Dennison teaches adults and children to do lazy eights to improve hand-eye coordination, promote efficient reading, and prevent eyestrain at the computer. A description of the lazy eights method appears in chapter 5.

Hands-on

These activities require that students use their hands to solve a problem or create a product that expresses what they have learned. A good example for high school algebra students is a game called "Wodjah and Company," described in Tim Erickson's *Get It Together*. Students work in groups using manipulatives to solve whimsical but challenging questions.

Kinesthetic Imagination

Yes, the muscles really can "imagine." Professional athletes have long been taught to enhance their practice by "seeing" themselves making a perfect pass or a three-point basket. More recently, they've been learning to "feel" themselves doing it while visualizing. There are more details later in this chapter. It's a natural for the classroom.

Perception Enhancement

We have more than five senses! When you're feeling tired, hungry, calm, stressed, or euphoric, you're experiencing several of the proprioceptive senses, the ones that perceive internally. *Experiencing these senses is a key to self-regulating behavior* and an important element in conflict resolution. Internal sensing and self-calming techniques are described later in this chapter.

A related enhancement activity is cross-sensing, or *synesthesia*. A great composer may "hear" a sunset and put it into music. Einstein "felt" insights about abstract concepts *in his muscles*. A cross-sensing technique is described in chapter 5.

Choose the Best Approach for Your Students

Should you be funny or straightforward? Should you use the kinesthetic activity as an introduction, as the core of a lesson, or as a follow-up? What kind of debriefing will you use? After a physical activity, it's wise to use a different modality to connect the activity with the more abstract aspects of the content. This connecting activity can consist of a written description of the learning, a diagram, a formula, a discussion, a picture, or even a song or a poem.

Can you give permission for students to participate in degrees, or do your students need more complete structure? I prefer to allow students to participate to the extent they feel comfortable, but I don't allow "wet blankets" or class clowns to disrupt the experience for others. Also, let students know that the ground rules for this kind of activity may differ from those for standard activities but that there are still rules. Following are some suggestions:

no put-downs

only positive feedback

no disruptive, destructive, or dangerous behavior

Sometimes it helps to use a consistent signal for this different learning modality: lowered lights or a particular kind of background music, for instance. Then when the lights are back to normal or the music is off, students understand that the regular ground rules are in operation again.

Explain Your Inclusion of Kinesthetic Activities (metacognitive learning)

If your students don't already know, tell them about their various intelligences, adapting the information from the introduction or using material specifically written for young people, such as *The*

Magic Seven by Nancy Margulies or *Seven Pathways of Learning* by David Lazear. Discussing the intelligences is a good way to help students become aware of their own learning processes. Moreover, it encourages them to sense themselves as partners in their own education, rather than as passive consumers—or worse, as victims. Essentially, it gives them an owner's manual for their own brains.

Once they know why they're using this approach to learning, students can begin to evaluate how well it serves them. This awareness helps them learn how to learn, an essential twenty-first century survival skill, since they're likely to need to change careers several times in their lifetimes. Someday we hope to develop cross-intelligent learners—those who can reconceptualize new information taught in other modalities into their own favored blend of intelligences. Metacognitive learning is a step in that direction.

Keep It Positive

If this kind of teaching is new for you, let students know that you're learning along with them. Our common body of knowledge, whether about subject matter or learning techniques, is constantly growing. Even the fields of science and math are changing focus as a result of deeper exploration by humanity's best minds. Recognize that some of your experiments in kinesthetic learning will work better than others.

Give students plenty of accurately detailed, positive feedback. Let the kinesthetic activities be as free from negative stress as possible, while you maintain appropriate limits on disruptive behavior.

Apply These Ideas to Assessment

Give students a chance to show what they know through projects, performances, and portfolios. They can make three-dimensional representations of concepts or design classroom games. They can use demonstrations, drama, pantomimes, and creative movement. They can create portfolios with photos of inventions, videotapes, and other multimedia products that show their understanding. David Lazear's book *Multiple Intelligence Approaches to Assessment* has dozens of good ideas.

Preliminary Skills Needed for Some of the Activities

In case you haven't already introduced your students to the many forms of active learning, this section suggests ways to prepare them. Not all the activities described in the chapters require these skills, but some may call for one or more of the following:

> *cooperative group work*
> *internal sensing (proprioception) and self-calming*
> *use of the kinesthetic imagination*
> *application of service learning to academic content*

Cooperative Group Work

Many teachers are already familiar with this approach, so I only touch on the basics. If your students are already experienced in cooperative learning, feel free to skip to the next section, "Internal Sensing and Self-Calming."

Declaration of Purpose

Explain that in the world of working adults, employers look for people who know how to work well with other people. These activities help students learn cooperative skills as well as subject matter.

Simple Warm-up Activities

If students are not familiar with one another, have them do a simple activity such as literary celebrity party (described in chapter 2) to become acquainted.

The One-Minute Move

Teach students to move quickly and quietly into groups within sixty seconds. This step may seem unnecessary, especially for high school juniors and seniors, but by making your expectations clear now, you save a great deal of time and frustration later. Ahead of time, randomly divide the class into pairs. Make another list of students randomly divided into groups of three to five.

To introduce the activity, tell students they will be doing some activities as partners and other activities in groups of three or more. Partners place their desks, touching, side by side or facing each other. For groups of more than two, each front corner of the desk should be touching the corner of another group member's desk. When students move their desks, they also need to move any other items they have brought to class, such as backpacks, books, and coats.

Announce the list of partners. Tell students that when you say, "Rumpelstiltskin!" (or any word you like), each set of partners will quietly move their desks so they're facing each other, get out a pencil and paper, and be ready within fifty-nine seconds, which gives them one second to breathe before you have them do the exercise again if they didn't all make it the first time. If they all make it, read the list of the larger groups and have students write down the names of the others in their group. Then give the starting signal again. Have students practice as often as necessary until they're reasonably efficient.

Other Guidelines

- Use positive body language and appropriate eye contact.
- Take turns talking and listening.
- Help one another. (It isn't cheating in this kind of activity.)
- Be tactful if you disagree.
- Stay on task.
- Be friendly; don't use put-downs; give positive comments.

Internal Sensing and Self-Calming

These skills are helpful for self-management, especially when students have the option of moving as they learn. Many young people have never paid much attention to their internal perceptions. For example, they may be restless, but not know it's because they had only a sugar doughnut for breakfast. Other students may pay a great deal of attention to the ups and downs of their insides, but have no concept of how to calm themselves and create their own sense of well-being. Following is an optional script for introducing internal sensing and self-calming, also called *centering*. A detailed description of centering and related activities is found in George Leonard's books, notably *Mastery* and *The Life We Are Given*, which he co-authored with Michael Murphy.

Optional Script

How many senses do we have? . . . Students generally say there are five. *Can you name some of them? . . .* Students usually list sight, hearing, touch, taste, and smell. *When you're feeling tired, which sense is that? . . . How about when you're energetic, hungry, or restless? These senses are internal, and we have lots of them. Some are inside the muscles and organs. Here's an example. Stand up next to your desk, without touching anything. Close your eyes and pay attention to what's helping you keep your balance.* Give students time to feel their balance. *The nerves in your muscles and your middle ear help you stay balanced. That exercise is a very simple example of internal sensing that goes on all the time. Thank you. Now sit down.*

Other internal senses are chemical. A tired or achy feeling after heavy exercise is partly a sense of the lactic acid in your muscles. Some people can sense when their blood sugar is low. Some people can even sense electrical changes in their brain waves. You probably already know that your brain sends out different kinds of electrical waves that can be measured with special equipment. Some people can learn what kinds of brain waves they're making and change them so they can think effectively or relax deeply, or be more creative.

In this class we won't go into brain waves, and you don't need to be preoccupied with your insides. Keep in mind, though, that you can often sense what's going on inside your body and you can make changes to help you feel better.

Have you ever tried calming yourself when you're restless, upset, or jittery? It isn't always easy, but I'll show you one way to do it, called centering. It's often used by martial artists, and sometimes by actors, athletes, and other individuals who are required to perform at a high level.

Before we start centering, I'd like you to practice just the opposite—being uptight. Stand next to your desks, very straight, feet together, shoulders back. Suck in your abdomen! Keep your eyes staring straight ahead, like a soldier at attention.

I'm going to give some of you a gentle shove on the shoulder and I'd like you to notice whether it's easy to keep your balance when you're standing stiff and straight like this.

Give light shoves to a few students—or all of them if it's feasible. Then let students relax while you ask them how it felt. Ask those who were shoved whether they were able to keep their balance easily.

Now I'd like to show you another way to stand. Put your feet a little apart—even with your shoulders. Your knees shouldn't be locked, but they shouldn't be bent either. Relax your stomach and, at the same time, keep your back and neck fairly straight. Pay attention to your shoulders. They aren't pulled back, but they're not slumped forward either. Breathe deeply and comfortably. Let the air move deep into you, all the way down into your abdomen. With your left hand, touch a spot just an inch or so below your navel. This is the center of gravity of your body. In Japanese martial arts such as karate and aikido, this center of gravity is sometimes called the hara. *We'll refer to it simply as your center.*

Keep breathing deeply and comfortably. Let your arms hang by your sides, nice and relaxed. Close your eyes. See if you can sense whether your weight is balanced evenly between your two feet. If you need to, shift a little from side to side until you find a good balance. Very gently, rock from front to back and find the place where your weight is evenly balanced between your heels and the balls of your feet. Keep your eyes closed and sense how it feels to be solidly balanced on your feet. Sometimes we refer to this state as being grounded. Please keep your eyes closed. Feel free to make a small shift to a more comfortable position if you need to.

Keep your eyes closed. Focus your attention on your spinal column—what we sometimes call your backbone. Sense the balance of each of the small bones in your spinal column, one on top of the other, working together to support your body and make it flexible. When you're centered, you only need a few muscles to keep your spinal column balanced; the rest can relax. Sense the bones in your neck, at the top of your spinal column. Move your head just a tiny bit from side to side and front to back until you find the place where it balances most easily on your neck. Let your attention go to the top of your head. Relax the muscles in your scalp and around your ears; in your forehead, your eyes, your cheeks; and around your mouth. Let go of any tightness in your jaw, your tongue, and your throat.

Put your attention on your shoulders. They're not pulled up tight, but they're not slumping forward either. They're just there at your sides, feeling relaxed like soft, warm chocolate. Keep breathing deeply and let that feeling of relaxation spread down your arms and into your hands and fingers. Let that warm chocolaty feeling spread down through your back and chest, your abdomen, your hips and thighs. Let it relax your legs and feet. Let yourself feel grounded and flexible, alert and relaxed. When you're balanced and centered, a lot of your muscles can be relaxed even when you're standing up.

Open your eyes for a moment. Keep breathing deeply and feeling what it's like to be centered and balanced. I'm going to give some of you another shove on the shoulder so you can notice if it's easier or harder to keep your balance this time. In a few minutes I'll ask you if you felt any difference. Give another gentle shove to the same students.

As you continue to breathe deeply and comfortably, close your eyes again. Let a beam of awareness go through your body, finding any places that don't feel relaxed and balanced. Sometimes that awareness by itself can help those tight places feel better.

Open your eyes now. Sit down gently at your desk. I hope you feel a bit more relaxed and alert at the same time. This exercise is one of the ways of getting centered and sensing what's going on inside you.

Lead a discussion of the activity. How did students feel when they were standing like soldiers? Did they feel different when they had gone through the centering process? Was it easier for students who were gently shoved to keep their balance when they were centered? Ask if they can think of any times when it would be especially useful to feel centered. (They might mention occasions such as before a big test, an important date, or a crucial game.)

As students are about to leave the class, have them take a minute to go through a brief repetition of the centering process.

Stand next to your desk again with your feet about shoulder width apart. Let your feet feel well balanced on the floor. Breathe deeply and comfortably, as if the breath can go all the way to your center. Let your belly and your back be relaxed but not slumping. Your arms are hanging comfortably at your sides. As you breathe, you feel as though your body and mind are balanced, relaxed, and alert. See if you can let this feeling stay with you for a while after you leave the class. If you lose it, you can come back to it whenever you want. To remind yourself how to do it, you can use the letters of the word grace. *Just remember to be*

> *grounded*
> > *relaxed*
> > > *aware*
> > > > *centered*
> > > > > *energized*

Have students practice self-calming often, especially before you give tests or introduce challenging material or activities.

Kinesthetic Imagination

Kinesthetic imagination is a form of muscular imagination, probably related to activity in the motor cortex of the brain, even though the body itself isn't necessarily moving. The kinesthetic imagination works with the visual and auditory imagination, so this kind of activity helps to integrate three or four intelligences.

Jean Houston's books give more detail on the use of this kind of imagination, calling it the "kinesthetic body" or the "imaginal body" (see bibliography). For details on athletes' use of the kinesthetic imagination, see Murphy (1992, 445).

Some of your students may already have this skill. If you teach the whole class to use the kinesthetic imagination, though, you are able to guide them on vivid imaginary journeys to places such as Shakespeare's England or the inside of an atom. This tool allows active involvement of the kinesthetic intelligence while students are sitting still. Here's an optional script for introducing the kinesthetic imagination.

Optional Script

Have you ever sat watching an impressive athlete or dancer perform on TV and felt as though you were performing, too? . . . Such a feeling is a form of muscular imagination. According to some scientists, it works because some of the nerves are active in the motor cortex of the brain, even though the body itself isn't moving. Some athletes and other individuals required to perform intensely use kinesthetic imagination to improve their skills. The athlete sees himself making a perfect basket and seems to feel it in his muscles at the same time, even though he's standing still. Then he tries it with his physical body and the shot is easier to make.

Maybe some of you already know how to use your kinesthetic imagination for things like this. If you don't already use this skill, you can start learning it with a few simple activities. If you're already familiar with it, you can extend your ability. Before we start, though, let's agree on one thing. For some of you, it may feel strange using your muscular imagination this way. If you feel uncomfortable with this activity, you don't have to participate, but you do need to be quiet and avoid disturbing anyone else.

Stand in a place where you're not touching anything. Breathe deeply and comfortably. Close your eyes to focus your awareness on the feelings in your muscles . . . With your right arm, reach straight up, as high as you can without straining. Stretch. Be aware of all the muscles in your arm, your hand, your fingers. Feel the other muscles that stretch as you hold your arm up . . .

Now put your arm down. Feel what it's like to relax all those muscles. Now raise the same arm again and feel all those muscles reaching and stretching. Lower your arm once more and feel the relaxation.

Now leave your right arm down but imagine that you're raising it, stretching it toward the ceiling. While your physical arm is at your side, your kinesthetic arm is reaching as high as it can. Imagine that you can feel all those muscles stretching . . . Now relax your kinesthetic arm and let it join your physical arm. Notice whether the muscles of that arm seem to be a bit more aware. Raise your physical arm again, but leave the kinesthetic arm down. How does it feel? Now slowly lower your physical arm and raise your kinesthetic one. See how it feels when one passes through the other.

Repeat the process with the left arm.

Now make sure there's enough space in front of you so you can jump about eight inches forward . . . Keep breathing deeply and comfortably. Be aware of the muscles in your whole body . . . Now make a small jump forward, just about eight inches. Let your muscles feel what it's like to make that jump . . . Jump back to where you started. Be aware of the muscles involved in jumping back . . . Now let your kinesthetic body jump forward while your physical body stays still . . . Feel those kinesthetic muscles . . . Let your kinesthetic body jump back into your physical body . . . Sit down now. How do you feel? . . .

Allow time for responses. If some students didn't feel anything, it's perfectly normal. Each person has different perceptions. Ask students simply to imagine that they're doing what you say. It's okay to pretend.

Now, while you're sitting still, let your kinesthetic body float up and walk on the ceiling. You can defy gravity with your kinesthetic body. Be careful not to bump into other kinesthetic bodies or trip on the light fixtures . . . Now let your kinesthetic body slide down the chalkboard or the wall, do a few flips in the air, then settle back into your physical body.

This kind of activity may seem strange in a classroom, but if it works for athletes, we can probably put it to use, too. We'll be using the kinesthetic imagination in other activities soon. Does anyone have more comments?

Allow for responses. If any students express discomfort or try to ridicule the idea, remind them that they don't have to participate in the activity, but they do need to be quiet and avoid disturbing anyone else.

Service Learning with Content

Service learning is largely a kinesthetic activity, and a very fruitful one. Following is an example.

A suburban middle school class visits a rural school in Appalachia, gets to know the host students, and together they study the health problems that may be caused by water pollution from the nearby paper mill. Would increased restrictions cause loss of jobs for local residents? Students undertake such projects as testing local water supplies, interviewing residents and businesspeople, and touring the paper mill. After a good deal of study and discussion, they make recommendations and contact their lawmakers. This kind of project provides active, kinesthetic involvement as well as application of learning in science, math, social studies, and English, while helping meet a need in a community.

Many people are talking about the values of service learning. Some school districts and state legislatures have instituted various service learning assignments as requirements for graduation. You may already have an active service learning program in your school. If so, you probably know how effective it can be for making academic learning meaningful.

If your school doesn't already have such a program, you might consider how to apply your subject specifically to community needs. This application gives students a direct, active use for the knowledge they're acquiring, and enhances the many other well-known benefits of service learning. Following are a few examples of applications.

English and Other Languages

- Students in an English class could team up with residents of a retirement home to write together about childhood memories, comparing their experiences and talking about the changes that have taken place over the years.

- Students in a foreign-language class could use their growing skill to help in bilingual classes.

- In connection with the study of *Romeo and Juliet*, students could volunteer at a teen suicide prevention agency. They wouldn't be expected to do the counseling that professionals do, but they could help with other chores to free the time of adults. Such assistance would give students a sense of participation and a deeper understanding of the needs of troubled teens and the value of intervention.

Social Sciences

- Civics students could help immigrants study for citizenship exams.
- History students studying the Depression could lend a hand in a program to feed the homeless.

Math and Natural Sciences

- Math students could tutor younger students or monitor traffic problems and suggest solutions based on time and motion studies.
- Biology students could volunteer at a health-care agency for the disadvantaged, or plant and maintain an on-campus garden.
- Chemistry students could monitor water pollution and suggest solutions.

Setting Up a Program in Service Learning

If your school doesn't already include a service learning component, here are some ways to initiate one. (The bibliography lists sources of information on service learning.) As in other new ventures, it may be wise to start small. Initially your project could be as simple as spending one class period doing something useful and relevant on campus. Such an approach keeps time and transportation requirements simple. If service learning is already required of students at your school, be sure to arrange your own project to fulfill students' obligations. Following are some suggested steps for conducting a service learning program:

1. Identify several community needs your class could address in the context of your subject. Take advantage of readily accessible information sources:
   - Browse newspapers.
   - Talk to colleagues on campus.
   - Ask community leaders and social agency personnel.

2. Estimate the resources required to meet these needs. (You don't have to solve the whole problem; just make a difference.)
   time
   transportation
   tools and supplies

3. Decide which need your class is capable of addressing. Involve students in the decision if possible. Be sure to clear your project with the appropriate administration and other authorities.

4. Structure the service project. At least for the first time, it may be best if the whole class works together under your supervision. Later, students might do service learning in small groups or individually, perhaps at different times and locations.

5. After completion of the project, notify the administration, student body, community (including parents), and the media about the success of the project so that students receive recognition for their efforts. Be sure to allow time for students to think, talk, write, or otherwise express their insights about the experience, including the satisfaction of feeling valued.

For further information on service learning, contact the National Youth Leadership Council or Youth Service America (see bibliography).

2 English and Other Languages

This chapter is divided into three sections: the first addresses literature, the next mechanics of language, and the third listening and speaking (primarily for second language teaching). Each section contains several suggested activities. At the end of the chapter is a sample text of an imaginary journey in literature.

Literature

Literature is fertile ground for active learning. The following activities are especially good for literature classes, although they have applications for other subjects as well, including written composition and second language learning.

Starters

These first two activities are useful to prepare the class for new works of literature.

Imaginary Journey in Literature

You can introduce a work of literature by taking students on an imaginary journey to the time and place of the story. Such imaging engages the kinesthetic imagination, described in chapter 1, as well as the visual, audial, and other senses. (For a sample script, see "Imaginary Journey in Literature: A Trip to Shakespeare's England" at the end of this chapter.)

Literary Celebrity Party

This activity is simple and can reinforce your introductory information on a new work of literature. Each student has a sign taped on her back listing a character's name, a place name, or a crucial item related to the plot. Students try to guess their celebrity identities by asking yes-no questions. The questioning can be done with one student in front of the class, in small groups, or as a whole-class activity, with students mingling and asking questions.

You can vary the game by letting each student know his own identity and having the others try to identify him using only yes-no questions. Students can mingle, trying to guess each person's identity then having each character sign a sheet of paper.

This activity can be used as a get-acquainted class warm-up, using names of well-known personalities. Each student receives a list of the personalities to find. As she guesses the identity of each, the "celebrity" writes his real name next to the celebrity's name on the list.

Informal Drama

An impersonation, a skit, a pantomime, or even a free-form dance can be a powerful tool in literature classes, serving to summarize the plot, to demonstrate or deepen students' understanding, or to act out alternative endings. You don't have to be an actor or drama coach yourself. No one is expecting professional quality; the purpose is to bring a taste of variety and to draw other intelligences into a primarily verbal discipline. When using informal dramatics in the classroom, be sure to give clear guidelines and time limits, both for preparation and for performance. If you wish, include costumes and props. (A box of hats, capes, and other evocative items is fun but not necessary.) In this section, I offer several simple dramatic activities then describe some more sophisticated uses of classroom dramatics.

Impersonations

Students focus on the characters in depth by doing individual impersonations, using simple props and costumes if you wish. An individual impersonator can introduce herself as the character, explain some of her motives at a given point in the story, and quote a few of her own lines, either from the text or in her own words. In the case of a shy student, the teacher can interview the character, asking simple "who, what, when, where" questions, leading to a possible "why" conclusion.

Group impersonations can include dialogues or arguments between characters, either in words from the text or in students' own paraphrasing. These encounters can occur between two characters from the same work, or two from different ones. For instance, what would Huckleberry Finn and *Cannery Row*'s Mack say to each other?

Getting into the Literary Picture

This activity adds color and drama to impersonations. Select a video of the piece of literature, choose a dramatic moment, and stop the action. Ask students to come to the front of the room and assume the same posture as the characters, using simple costumes and props if you wish. You can interview each of them about their actions and motivations, or they can carry on a dialogue in their own words about the issues portrayed in the scene (see figure 2-1).

Another version of this technique, suggested in the *History Alive!* program developed by Teachers' Curriculum Institute (see bibliography), involves projecting a slide of an illustration from the book. The *History Alive!* materials provide a richly detailed outline of this technique, which they call the interactive slide lecture. The outline includes suggested methods for making slides from book illustrations. See chapter 3 for more details.

Raps

Tapes of the toe-tapping "Romeo and Juliet Rap" and "Julius Caesar Rap" are available from Teachers' Discovery (see bibliography). To get students physically involved while they listen, have them do something as simple as tapping pencils on their desks or as active as getting up and

Chapter 2

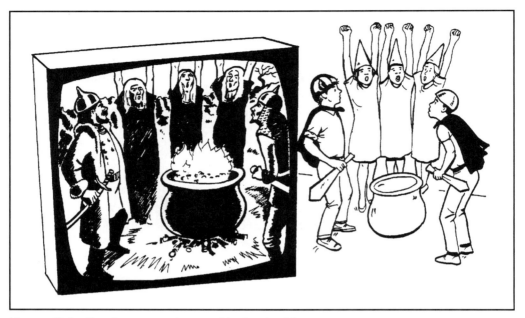

Figure 2-1. Students get into a *Macbeth* video

dancing. Since the tapes come with written lyrics, students can later present them as lip-synch dramas, perform them using their own voices and instruments, or make up entirely new raps. Students who like to compose raps can tailor them to virtually any subject area.

Kinesthetic Shakespeare for All Levels

Informal classroom drama has been used effectively to teach Shakespeare to elementary through university levels (Patterson 1989; Flachmann 1996). I've personally had great success using informal drama for the introduction of Shakespeare's works to elementary and middle school students. First, students do activities and puzzles, including an imaginary journey, to gain familiarity with Shakespeare's England, Elizabethan language, the background of the plot, and the characters. Then, using shortened but authentic texts, students read the play in dramatic form (one student as Romeo, another as Juliet, and so on). If possible, they also watch a video of the play and "get into the picture" in several key scenes. After an appropriate written follow-up, students launch into "theatrical frolics," reader's theater performances of key scenes, using simple props and costumes. This exercise delves into some of the deep human issues of the plays, including internal and external temptation in *Macbeth*, manipulation in *Julius Caesar*, distinguishing justice from revenge in *Romeo and Juliet* and *The Merchant of Venice*, dealing with suicidal thoughts in *Hamlet*, and conflict resolution in all the plays. (The conflict resolution techniques outlined in chapter 5 can be applied to the teaching of Shakespeare and most other good literature.)

Michael Flachmann, Carnegie Foundation Professor of the Year for 1995, uses informal dramatics to teach Shakespeare to his university students. Many of his techniques, which we discussed in several conversations during February and March 1996, are applicable to middle and high school classes and are detailed in a forthcoming book. Flachmann contends that Shakespeare was meant to be staged, not just read silently, so he often introduces aspects of stagecraft. In focusing his students' attention on a particular scene, for example, he has them decide how they would block it (show how characters would enter, stand, move, and interact). Reading the lines and moving appropriately within a "stage" area, students develop a deeper understanding and longer memory of the dynamics of the piece. Actors sometimes talk of "body memory," saying that they can memorize their lines more effectively once the blocking is done.

In an activity called "Paraphrase and Subtext," Flachmann has three students line up one behind the other. The first reads certain lines from the script. The second student paraphrases the lines in contemporary English. The third student narrates what actors call the "subtext," discussing the characters' thoughts, feelings, and hidden motivations, which may be very different from the spoken words.

Flachmann might ask a student posing as King Lear to describe Lear's dysfunctional family in Act I and again in Acts III and V. Perhaps the Earl of Kent would join the conference and give his comments. Sometimes Flachmann has characters from different plays interact, asking such questions as "How would Hamlet and Othello have reacted if their situations were reversed?" He points out that in a sense, all Shakespeare's characters exist within us; each of us houses the qualities of Iago, Brutus, Desdemona, Nick Bottom, Lady Macbeth, and others. The same can probably be said of the major characters in all great literature. Kinesthetic activities offer students a means of identifying these elements in themselves, thereby cultivating a deeper understanding of the literary work, of their own being, and of the human condition.

Follow-up: Three-Dimensional Models or Dioramas

To culminate the study of a work of literature, students can construct models or dioramas of the setting, a dramatic scene, or a sequence of events. Students can use a wide range of materials, from cardboard to ceramic clay, and they can do the projects either individually or in small groups. You may need to give size guidelines, as a group of enthusiastic builders can easily use a great deal of space.

Mechanics of Language

Many people think that the mechanical aspects of language must be taught with plenty of pencil-and-paper drills or oral repetition while students sit in one place. This method works well to some extent, but you also have the choice of using plenty of lively strategies that engage the bodily-kinesthetic intelligence.

Spelling, Vocabulary, Verb Forms, and Writing Systems

Following are some ways to breathe life into the sometimes tedious practice that students need with individual words.

Sign Language Alphabet

The American Sign Language alphabet can be helpful in unexpected ways, even to students who can hear well. Years ago I had a student who did well in everything but spelling. She happened to learn the sign language alphabet and found that she could memorize irregular words by spelling them out with the manual alphabet. The same technique can facilitate learning of vocabulary, scientific terminology, and other items that need to be memorized. (See figure 2-2 for the sign language alphabet.)

Write on What??
Students who have difficulty learning an unfamiliar writing system can practice writing in huge letters, using the whole arm rather than just the hand. This type of writing can be scrawled on the chalkboard, scratched in sand on the ground, or even traced on the back of a fellow student, who tries to recognize the letter or word.

Picture Derby
Try this method as a vocabulary review. Divide the class into two teams. Each team chooses its first contestant, who goes to the chalkboard. The teacher silently shows a word to the first two contestants, who each try to draw a picture to represent the word as their teams watch. A point goes to the team that guesses the word first. The game continues with other students drawing until students have adequately reviewed all the words.

Vocabulary Charades
Students work individually or in small groups to play charades with vocabulary words. Before starting, the class agrees on hand signals to indicate the part of speech and gender (if applicable). Students can represent the number of syllables by holding up the corresponding number of fingers. The student then acts out the meaning, and the class tries to guess the word.

Verb Form or Noun Declension Charades
This charade is more complex but is very effective for reviewing verb forms. The class first agrees on conventional signals to represent the person, number, and tense of the

Chapter 2

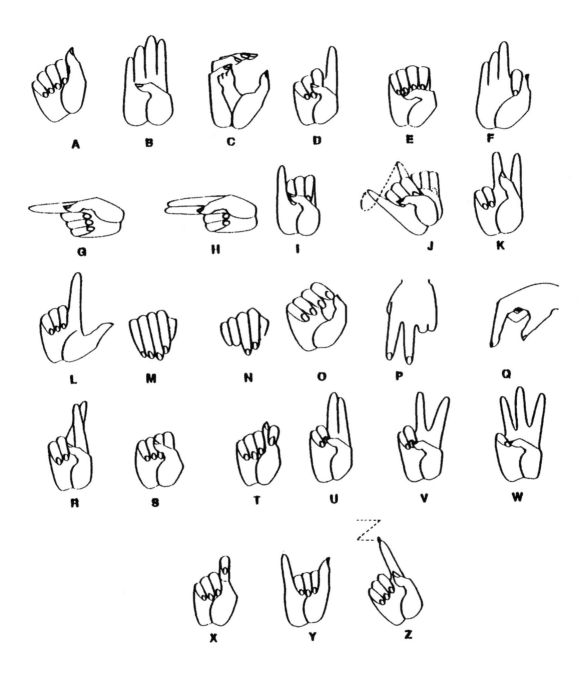

Figure 2-2. American Sign Language manual alphabet

verb form. (For example, the student points to himself to indicate the first person singular, or to himself and another person for the first person plural. He may point backward to indicate the past tense and forward for the future.)

The class divides into teams; students take turns as the presenter. The presenter gives the hand signs for person, number, and tense, then acts out the meaning of the verb. Each team sends a contestant to write the correct verb form on the board as quickly as possible. Contestants must take turns, but team members can quietly help the contestant to remember the correct form. That way, everyone participates, and students receive help in a playful context. Depending on your preference, the contestant may or may not be allowed to take to the board a paper with the form written on it. You can use the same technique to review cases of nouns or adjectives in languages such as German or Latin.

Sentence, Paragraph, or Essay Structure

Putting words together effectively requires a good deal of practice, a process you can enliven with kinesthetic activities.

Punctuation Sounds and Actions

For each punctuation mark, the class can decide on a gesture and an appropriately goofy sound. A period, for example, can be represented by pointing one finger forward while whistling a single tone. Two fingers pointing forward and two whistles, one lower than the other, can signal a colon. After a little practice, the class can read aloud unpunctuated passages, supplying the necessary punctuation gestures and sounds. There will be lots of laughs, but plenty of effective review of punctuation.

Michael Flachmann described a more active variation of this activity to me. Flachmann's variation has oversized punctuation marks taped onto the chests of students. Each student is asked to decide on an appropriate way of impersonating that particular punctuation mark. As a passage is read aloud, the "punctuation people" jump up as needed.

Sentence Ad-Libs

For this review of sentence structure, divide the class into teams. Each team has one person or subgroup responsible for the subject and a subgroup responsible for the predicate. The predicate group has one person select the verb, another the direct object, and so on, depending on the sentence structure you select. The teams take turns constructing clever sentences with the subject subgroup making up the subject, the verb person adding a verb, and so on through the sentence. Encourage students to make the sentences as funny as possible. Team 2 takes its turn, and the game continues until all students have participated. You can vary the sentence structure infinitely to provide drills in various constructions. Once students are accustomed to this kind of ad-lib, you can ask them to act out the words instead of saying them, having the rest of the class guess the meaning of the sentence.

Paragraph or Essay Ad-Libs

In this variant of the preceding activity, team members meet for a few minutes to help one another make up their sentences. Then, taking turns, one team member gives the topic sentence of a paragraph, others give the supporting sentences, and a final person gives the closing sentence. If you wish, you can supply the topic sentences for each team. To review essay structure, follow a similar procedure. One person gives the thesis sentence, others supply the supporting paragraphs, and a final member provides the conclusion.

Listening and Speaking Skills

These activities are primarily for second-language classes, where the body can effectively enhance the work of the ears and the mouth.

Total Physical Response (TPR)

More and more teachers are beginning to use the approach called *total physical response,* developed by James J. Asher and widely taught by the respected presenter Berty Segal. I summarize the approach here. For more details, see Asher 1993, Segal 1995, and Krashen and Terrell 1983.

The approach is based on the observation that children learn their first language by *listening* to the adults around them. Long before they can speak, babies and toddlers generally show a surprising degree of comprehension. And those babies are not just learning a second language; they're constructing the entire concept of verbal communication! While babies are going through this process, no one expects the little tykes to speak with perfect pronunciation, to read words, or to take notes. There are no tests or grades, and babies usually receive a huge amount of positive feedback with each little accomplishment.

As scientists studied how babies acquire language, they found that a large percentage of what the babies heard from parents and caregivers was in the form of commands: "Give Mommy a smile!" "Open your mouth wide," or "Run to Daddy." Even before knowing how to talk, a toddler can often follow a series of commands: "Pick up your red truck, put it in your toy box, and come and get a cookie." The researchers found that most babies' environments are low stress, the parents' communications are understandable and often accompanied by visual cues, and the child has plenty of time to hear and respond nonverbally before being expected to talk.

Asher and others advocate an approach to second language learning that more nearly approximates the way that children acquire their first language. Students begin simply hearing commands in the new language, such as *stand, sit,* or *walk*. As teachers give these commands, they model them and have the class imitate the actions. Soon students are able to follow the commands without needing the teacher to model them. As the teacher gives new commands, it is often possible to combine them with old ones in a humorous way. For example, after the teacher has introduced the command "Put your book on the table," she might say, "Put your foot on the table." This approach allows for endless lighthearted drills that involve physical action, targeting information storage in long-term rather than in short-term memory.

Within six to twelve lessons, depending on age, students spontaneously start giving the commands themselves, showing that they are ready to talk rather than just to listen and respond. The physical activities can continue throughout the course of language learning, as students also learn to read and write the language (preferably using highly motivating materials). A number of studies have documented the efficacy of the TPR approach (for example, Asher 1993). Berty Segal and James Asher offer a wide variety of teaching materials in this approach. (See the entries in the English and Second Languages section of the bibliography.)

More Activities for Listening and Speaking

In this section are examples of physical activities that have worked well with second and third-year high school students. They were done originally in a Spanish class but are described in English so they can be adapted to any second language class.

"Baking" Cookies

Even jaded and bored adolescents seem to thrive on this activity. You don't need an oven, and you won't make a mess in the classroom. Students only pantomime the cookie baking actions, but you still need a recipe, some props, and enough real cookies for the whole class. Following is a summary of the steps:

1. Translate a simple recipe for chocolate chip cookies into the target language. Make a copy for each student. Gather the ingredients. (You won't actually mix them. You can even use empty packages.)

2. Collect utensils: mixing bowl and spoons, measuring cups and measuring spoons, and at least two cookie sheets.

3. On the day of the lesson, fill one cookie sheet with the real cookies you've brought. Put it into a cabinet or other appropriate place that represents the oven. Be sure there's room in the "oven" for another cookie sheet, which comes later.

4. Explain in the target language that students are going to help you bake cookies. Distribute the copies of the recipe. As students read it to you, point to each ingredient, then pantomime the actions of preparing the cookie dough and spooning it onto the cookie sheet.

5. After this demonstration, ask for a pair of volunteers to mix another batch of imaginary cookie dough. Have class members read the instructions as the volunteers pantomime the process of measuring, mixing, and dolloping the imaginary dough on the cookie sheet.

6. Put the cookie sheet into the "oven." After a few minutes, during which you review the target vocabulary or grammatical structures, take out the sheet of real cookies and pass them around.

Vocabulary includes such words as *measure, add, mix, stir, bake, cool, spoonful, cupful, flour, sugar, salt, chocolate,* and *nuts.* Grammatical structures include command forms, passive voice, and subjunctive.

Restaurant

The purpose of this activity is to introduce or review restaurant vocabulary and to give students confidence in one of the essential survival skills in a new language: ordering food in a restaurant. Materials needed are sample menus in the target language, and props for the "restaurant": napkins, plates, glasses, cups, saucers, spoons, forks, knives, tablecloth, candles, flower vases, and so on.

As preparation, groups of class members review restaurant vocabulary by looking at several examples of menus, then writing their own. The class is divided into groups of restaurateurs and groups of customers. The restaurateurs take turns setting the table and preparing for the customers. One or more serve as waiters. The customers enter and are seated. They read the menu, order, and chat while the waiter brings the food. The customers comment on the food, ask for the bill, pay, and say good-bye to the restaurateurs. It may take several restaurant skits to give the whole class an opportunity to practice, but the activity can be varied by choosing different kinds of menus from among those students have written.

Magic Lamp

This skit helps students practice using command forms or practice subjunctive forms by using such phrases as "I want that you . . . " or "I would like that you . . . " The spoken roles are for the Narrator, the Lucky Protagonist, and the Genie. It helps to have a small brass lamp or bowl as a prop.

Narrator	*You are walking on the beach. You see something shiny in the sand. You pick it up. It is an ancient brass lamp. You rub it to clean off the sand, and suddenly a genie appears! (The Lucky Protagonist and Genie act out this scenario during the narration.)*
Genie	*A thousand thanks, O Wise One! You have saved me from the curse of an evil magician. You may make three wishes, and I will make them come true. Tell your servant what your three wishes are.*

The Lucky Protagonist, following the structure given by the teacher, utters his three wishes. As with the restaurant activity, students can repeat this dialogue as often as necessary to give several students practice.

Blind Date

Based on the Dating Game TV game show, this rather advanced activity provides lighthearted but structured conversation. (In Spanish, the program is "Cita con el Amor.") The master of ceremonies introduces a young man to the audience. On the other side of a partition, visible to the audience but not to the young man, are three or more young ladies who are potential dates. The young man asks each young woman one or two questions (samples follow), then he must choose his date sight unseen. After he makes his choice, the master of ceremonies introduces the lucky young woman, then announces a wonderful or ridiculous place where the happy couple will go for their date, courtesy of several imaginary sponsors.

In the next portion of the show or with the next group, a young woman asks questions of several young men and chooses one as her date, according to the same procedure.

Following are some sample questions for the "date" to ask:

- What makes a couple get along well?
- What would you do if I didn't show up for our first date?
- What do you do to make a good impression on a woman?
- What do you think would be the ideal date?
- If you could do something positive for the world, what would it be?
- If your boyfriend is busy and can't pay much attention to you, what do you do?
- If you had to be a caterpillar tractor, a roller skate, or a milk shake, which would you choose? Why?

Superwhammo

Students work in small groups to invent a "product" called Superwhammo (or another name if they prefer). They make a prototype, devise a visual advertisement for it, and present a radio or television commercial, all in the target language, of course. The commercial can be done as a skit, an audiotape, or a videotape.

Chapter 2

Sample Script: Imaginary Journey in Literature

A Trip to Shakespeare's England

Climb into your imagination and go with me to England as it was about four hundred years ago. Close your eyes for a while and we'll leave behind our cars, telephones, refrigerators, electric lights, television, computers, and stereos. We'll also leave behind our nuclear weapons, acid rain, CFCs, and drug problems.

Imagine that we're walking along a muddy country road. Let your feet feel what it's like to walk on the squishy roadbed. It's a sunny morning with scattered clouds in a blue sky and a bracing April breeze. You feel an occasional drop of water falling from the leaves of overhanging trees. It rained yesterday and it may rain again before we reach London. Your muscles stretch as we quicken our pace.

We reach the King's Highway, which is also mostly mud, with occasional stretches of rough paving stones. There are a few carts and carriages lumbering along through the ruts and puddles, but it's a bumpy and treacherous ride for them. Most people either walk or ride horses. We notice a heavy carriage mired up to its hubs in a puddle. Four footmen are straining to push while the coachman urges the horses to pull it out. A stocky gentleman in black velvet stands by, shouting at the coachman. You see a few logs of dead wood nearby, and with the help of the rest of us, you jam them under the wheels. As the coach begins to lurch forward, one footman neglects to shift his weight and sprawls face-first in the mud. His fellow servants give him a good teasing and help him up as the gentleman's valet thanks us graciously and gives each of us three pennies: the price of a good meal in a London inn.

We travel on through the green countryside dotted with farms, woods, and occasional country mansions. The road is getting more crowded. Peasants in rough homespun clothes brush against us, herding calves or sheep to market. Be careful of what you step in. Tradesmen pass by, some on foot, others on horses. We hear galloping hoofbeats behind us and scramble out of the way just in time to avoid being splattered with mud by a royal messenger.

At length we pass through the gates of London. We walk down the crowded, bumpy cobblestone streets, listening to vegetable sellers and fish-vendors calling for buyers. Passing a kitchen, we smell bread baking. We still have to be careful where we step; the streets are none too clean. There are no sewers, no garbage collectors, and no indoor plumbing in Shakespeare's London. People dump garbage and waste water that runs down the ditch at the center of the street. Maids empty chamber pots out of second-story windows. Watch out! There's one now! A quick move just saves you from getting doused with something smelly.

Hearing a huge clamor ahead, we see a grand procession of lords and ladies wearing velvets and silks. Six or eight lords are carrying a litter with a throne on it. On the throne is Her Majesty, Queen Elizabeth herself. She wears a magnificent white silk gown with a high ruffled collar, heavily embroidered and decorated with pearls. Her red hair also has strands of pearls woven through it. We bow deeply as she passes, and as we look up, she waves. You feel a shiver of excitement. A cheer rises from the throats of her subjects, "Long live good Queen Bess!"

Crossing London Bridge, we walk to a large, round, wooden building with a flag flying at the top. This is the Globe Theater, where we can pay a penny to go in and see the play. Of course, a penny only gives us space to stand on the ground in the center of the round theater with the boisterous young apprentices and others who can't afford to buy a seat. We jostle around among these groundlings for a moment, then spend a few more pence for a reasonably comfortable spot on a bench, a little above the groundlings. As we sit and rest our tired bones, we can see the lords and fine ladies taking their cushioned seats. A play by the well-known playwright Will Shakespeare is about to begin. It's a murder mystery featuring a ghost, a king and queen, a brooding young prince, swashbuckling sword fights, and a bit of comedy to make the groundlings laugh.

Not far away, a fight breaks out between a burly miller and a pair of arrogant soldiers. People start screeching and running in all directions. We try to move out of the way as the miller tosses the two soldiers like flour sacks right into our laps. Our

Chapter 2

bench tips over backward. We feel like we'll be smothered or trampled, but instead we're being swirled around through space and time. Suddenly we come to a stop. Opening our eyes, we find ourselves back in our classroom, remembering our eventful trip to Shakespeare's London.

Now, quietly write a paragraph, draw a picture, or plan a skit, pantomime, or dance to describe your experience in Shakespeare's England.

3 Social Sciences

You can integrate a cornucopia of activities into social science classes to make the subject matter come alive. I talk about history first, then about geography and economics.

History

As in other subjects, in history classes you can integrate kinesthetic activities that are either very simple or quite elaborate. I start with a few simple ones, then go on to describe some activities that simulate personal participation in historical events.

Simple Starters

Human Graph

Because graphs are so commonly used in historical materials, it's sometimes helpful to have students experience becoming a bar graph by standing in lines that express class distribution of certain characteristics. Introductory human graphs can show how many students were born in your state or in other states or countries. Human graphs dramatize such historical factors as the approximate number of British regulars compared to the number of minutemen at various stages of the Battles of Lexington and Concord.

Human Continuum

Whenever an issue in the class invites a wide range of possible opinions, you can ask students to express their opinions by getting out of their seats and arranging themselves along a line that serves as a continuum from one extreme to the other.

Following is an example.

Assume you're studying issues that divided the United States shortly before World War I. At one end of the chalkboard, write the word *Isolationist.* At the other end, write the word *Imperialist.* In the middle, write *Interventionist.* Ask students to imagine that they're United States senators just before World War I. After a short discussion of the terms of the policies and their relevance to the period, ask students to make a preliminary decision on what policy they would support. Then have them get up and stand in front of the chalkboard to show their positions, isolationist, interventionist, imperialist, or somewhere in between. Students may be bunched in one particular part of the continuum or they may be widely distributed. Some may be contrarians, expressing an opinion that most others would disagree with just to spark debate. Rather than creating a disruption, such dissension breathes life into a class discussion.

It's often helpful to do this activity at the very beginning of a lesson, explaining to students that they're free to change their minds as they learn more about the issue. That's part of what learning is all about. Repeating the activity at the end of the lesson dramatizes the value of delving deeply into an issue and considering all sides of it.

The next few activities may sound familiar. They were described in chapter 2 in relation to English or second language classes and are applied here to history.

Imaginary Journey in History

Your students can experience a moment in history by taking an imaginary journey that invokes the kinesthetic, visual, auditory, and other senses. For a sample script, see "Escape from Srebrenica" at the end of this chapter.

Historical Celebrity Party

Follow the same instructions as in the chapter 2 literary celebrity party. The celebrities in your history class can be historical characters, events, or even issues or trends.

Informal Dramatics

Skits, pantomimes, and free-form dance are splendid cooperative activities. Nearly any historical event can be portrayed dramatically, and students can explore alternative resolutions. You only need to give clear guidelines on preparation and performance time, and space available. Costumes and props are optional. If students have a bit of traditional mime training, props aren't usually necessary. (For information on the use of mime in the classroom, see the bibliography listings on Gail Herman and Patricia Hollingsworth, and Richard Shope.)

Impersonations

Students do individual impersonations, using costumes and props if desired, representing specific characters or types, such as a 1918 suffragette. In pairs or groups, they can stage debates or discussions, personifying representatives of various viewpoints. Some possibilities follow:

> Athenians and Spartans in 427 B.C.E.
>
> Richard the Lionhearted and Philip II of France in C.E. 1191
>
> Patriots and Loyalists in C.E. 1774

Getting into the Historical Picture

Embody a historical event or issue by using a video portraying the event and stopping it at a dramatic point. Have several volunteers stand in front of the scene and, if possible, get into the positions of the people represented (some may need to change position after a while). You can interview each student in the picture as if she were that historical character and let students discuss their points of view. For a variation of this activity, see the description of the interactive slide lecture in the *History Alive!* program, later in this chapter.

Historical Zingers (More Elaborate, but Worth the Effort)

Inventing the U.S. Government

In this activity, students work either individually or in small groups to assume the identity of one person who was influential at the Constitutional Convention. After researching the individual's life and political position, students read one or more accounts of the Constitutional Convention, taking notes on that individual's role. (For younger students, I recommend Jean Fritz's book *Shh! We're Writing the Constitution!*) Following is a chart of possible characters:

Constitutional Characters		
George Washington	Virginia	Although strongly in favor of a strong central government, he was wise enough to know that as president of the convention, he could not express any preferences.
Patrick Henry	Virginia	Famous for his revolutionary speech ending with "Give me liberty or give me death!" he totally opposed the idea of a strong central government, boycotted the convention, and campaigned tirelessly against ratification in his state of Virginia, once giving eight speeches in one day. Nevertheless, his fellow Virginians overruled him. He was influential, however, in supporting the addition of the Bill of Rights.

Alexander Hamilton	New York	A brilliant, controversial political thinker, he strongly favored strong national government and wrote most of the *Federalist Papers*, which helped persuade many people to support ratification. He became the first secretary of the Treasury, created the Bank of the United States, and established credit for the new nation at home and abroad. In 1800 he caused a rift in the Federalist Party by opposing the reelection of John Adams. He supported his old political rival, Thomas Jefferson, against Aaron Burr, who lost the election. In 1804 a duel between Burr and Hamilton resulted in Hamilton's death.
John Jay	New York	Another strong Federalist, he helped write the *Federalist Papers* and later became the first chief justice of the Supreme Court. In 1794 he negotiated a treaty with England that averted a war over English interference with American shipping. Jay's treaty established a base for the new nation's economic prosperity.
James Madison	Virginia	Sometimes called the Father of the Constitution, he took copious notes throughout the convention, which have been helpful over the centuries in helping interpret the Constitution. He was another of the writers of the *Federalist Papers* and later became the fourth president of the United States.
Benjamin Franklin	Pennsylvania	The oldest delegate at 81 years, he sometimes fell asleep during sessions, but his unfailing humor and legendary wisdom helped to keep the convention on track and to convince reluctant delegates to sign the final document.

Edmund Randolph	Virginia	Governor of Virginia as well as representative to the convention, he presented the Virginia Plan, which introduced the idea of three branches of government. The executive branch would be in charge of running the government. The legislative branch, Congress, would make the laws and would consist of a House of Representatives elected by the people and of a smaller body, the Senate, to be elected by the House of Representatives. The third branch would be the judicial branch, and it would ensure the constitutionality of the laws. Ironically, when the Constitution was in its final form, very similar to Randolph's plan, he refused to sign it. He wanted more protection of individual and state rights. He supported ratification in the Virginia legislature, however. Later he defended Aaron Burr in his trial for treason.
William Paterson	New Jersey	He presented the New Jersey Plan, which opposed Randolph's Virginia Plan. This plan preserved the loose confederation, gave each state an equal vote in a unicameral legislature, and called for a group of executives to head the government. At one point during the acrimonious debate, he and other representatives of small states threatened to secede and form their own confederation.

Roger Sherman	Connecticut	He proposed the "Great Compromise," calling for equal representation in the Senate, balanced by representation according to population in the House. This compromise saved the convention from disintegrating and established the basis for the present government.
Elbridge Gerry	Massachusetts	He was sometimes called the "Grumbletonian." He strongly opposed the Virginia Plan, and at the last minute refused to sign the Constitution although his fellow Massachusetts delegates agreed with it. Later, as governor of Massachusetts, he had the dubious honor of giving his name to the term "gerrymander" when he attempted to manipulate electoral districts in his party's favor.
Gouverneur Morris	Pennsylvania	He had aided the patriot cause during the Revolution and assisted with the new nation's finances. He was one of the best speakers at the convention. During the deliberations on the number of years of citizenship required for election to federal office, he pointed out that if it took seven years to learn to be a shoemaker, a foreigner should be required to spend fourteen years as a citizen learning to be an American lawmaker. (The convention finally settled on seven years for a representative and nine for a senator.)

Chapter 3

John Rutledge	South Carolina	He had served as governor of South Carolina during the chaotic Revolutionary War years. In the Constitutional Convention, he unsuccessfully pushed for a property ownership requirement as a qualification for holding office. He favored continuation of slavery and the division of society into classes as a basis for representation. After the convention's concessions to southern states, he strongly supported the Constitution. Rutledge later became an associate justice of the Supreme Court. He was nominated as chief justice in 1795, but the Senate refused to confirm the nomination.

- Students should research the figure's background.

  the person's upbringing and any important accomplishment made before 1787

  the person's stand on strong central government (Patrick Henry, for example, was strongly against it. He boycotted the convention, but his influence was important.)

  the person's economic orientation: agricultural, business, patrician, and so on

  the person's state population (small or large)

  the person's stand on slavery

  the person's suggestions that ultimately became part of the Constitution

  the person's stand on the Bill of Rights

  the person's final stand on ratification

  the person's important accomplishments after 1789

- Students should find out the problems with the Articles of Confederation that caused some statesmen to think changes were needed (sample answers follow):
    - Congress had sole authority to govern.
    - Each state had one vote.
    - Nine votes were needed to enact laws.
    - A unanimous vote was required to amend the Articles of Confederation.
    - A weak executive committee was to oversee government when Congress was out of session.
    - No national court system was instituted.
    - States could refuse to contribute funds to run government.
    - States printed their own money, of dubious value.
    - The United States was so weak that its independence was in danger.
- Students should find out about the discomfort the delegates faced at the convention.
    - heat and flies
- Students should find out about dilemmas the delegates faced.
    - whether they should establish a strong central government
    - whether the head of government might become a tyrant
    - whether the president should be elected for life
- Students should research the qualifications required of candidates.
    - whether it should be possible to remove the president from office
    - whether the nation should abolish slavery

Chapter 3

> whether large states should have more representatives than small ones

whether the nation needed a Bill of Rights

- Students should find out the factors that contributed to success of the convention and the ratification effort (sample answers follow):

  > decision to keep deliberations secret

  George Washington's prestige and scrupulous neutrality

  > Ben Franklin's sense of humor

  presence of some fine political thinkers who had the courage to draw on ideas of Locke, Rousseau, and Montesquieu

  > Virginia Plan (three branches) proposed by Edmund Randolph

  "Great Compromise" (equal representation in Senate and representation according to population in House) proposed by Roger Sherman

  > balance of power, emphasized by Hamilton, Madison, and Jay

  agreement to add the Bill of Rights

- Students should find out what kind of government the group invented.
- Students should discover the ways in which it differed from governments of other countries at the time.

After doing their research, the group can write a report including all information. Later, each group can be featured in one of the following activities:

- A soliloquy on some constitutional question. For example, George Washington might talk about how important a strong central government is, and how difficult it is to remain scrupulously neutral as president of the convention.

Social Sciences

- A debate with one or more other characters. For example, William Paterson might insist on the rights of small states, championing equal representation in Congress for each state. In contrast, Edmund Randolph might insist on representation according to population. Roger Sherman could solve the disagreement by proposing the "Great Compromise." (See figure 3-1.)

- A "Meet the Press" style interview in which the character is asked pointed questions by other characters.

For any of these activities, students need to defend the character's political position as well as possible. You can heighten interest by using costumes, props, and visual aids.

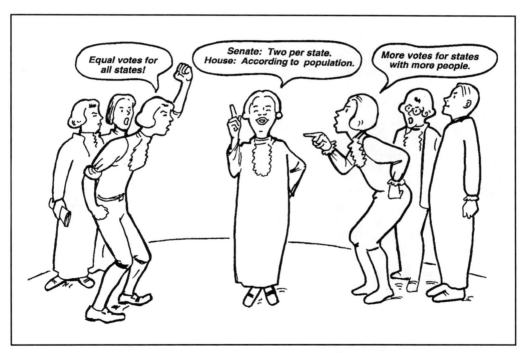

Figure 3-1. Students play delegates to Constitutional Convention

Amendment Boogie

Assign students to groups in which to research the amendments to the Constitution. Each group prepares a skit, rap, or dance to demonstrate the meaning of each and how it relates to the others. In their productions, students may use appropriate visual aids, props, and costumes to communicate the following information.

> the reasons the amendment was needed
>
> the date the amendment was proposed
>
> the content of the amendment in students' own words
>
> the date the amendment was ratified
>
> the effects of the amendment on the nation.

You may group the amendments according to their main emphases:

> basic individual and states' rights: 1-10, 11, 13
>
> right to vote: 14, 15, 19, 23, 24, 26
>
> elections, terms, and taxes: 12, 16, 17, 20, 22, 25
>
> alcohol: 18, 21

Highlights from *History Alive!*

The *History Alive!* program from Teachers' Curriculum Institute is geared toward students with various learning styles. It allows them to work in cooperative groups and to experience history rather than just sit through a lecture or plow through a textbook. Its techniques are designed for middle school and high school classes and can be applied to a wide range of historical topics. The overall program is described in a single volume called *History Alive!* which is accompanied by a professional development video program. In addition, Teachers' Curriculum Institute offers detailed lesson plans for several levels (see bibliography). Here I describe some of the activities especially relevant to kinesthetic learning.

Interactive Slide-Lecture

To make a period of history come alive, project a slide of a dramatic scene from the period under study. Ask students to describe in detail what they see. Students then get up and assume the positions of characters in the picture and tell the story from their own points of view. *History Alive!* gives a wealth of practical details on this technique. Especially helpful are the suggestions for making slides from book illustrations.

Experiential Activities

These activities usually last for one class period and help students experience something similar to the event or conditions of the targeted period. In one activity students experience the stress of working on an assembly line. Students place their desks side-by-side in two rows that face each other. Each row of students mass-produces copies of a drawing of a person. Each student draws a single part of the person, then passes the paper on quickly to the next participant until the drawing is finished. The teacher acts as the "boss," demanding faster, better work. Some teachers make the room uncomfortably hot or dim the lights to make the environment resemble a sweat shop. After this simulation, students have a deeper understanding of the conditions in the factories of the industrial revolution and, in some cases, modern times. (See figures 3-2 and 3-3.)

In another activity, "Reliving the Trenches of World War I," students huddle in trenches made of desks and chairs, listening to passages that describe life in the trenches. Later they write letters describing the experience.

Students participating in a third activity, "Re-creating the Paranoia of 1950s McCarthyism," each have a piece of paper that secretly identifies them as "acceptable" or "unacceptable." The acceptable ones try to form as large a group as possible, but must determine acceptability without seeing other students' papers. Both groups experience the effects of unfounded suspicion and guilt by association.

Chapter 3

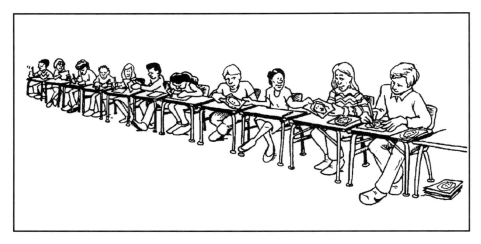

Figure 3-2. Students simulate working on an assembly line

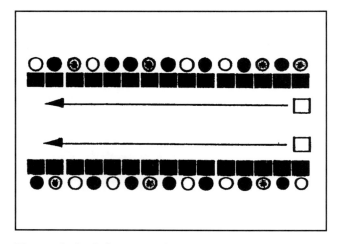

Figure 3-3. Schematic for assembly line

Historical Museum

Assign groups of students to create a museum with at least four exhibits that represent the historical period under study and that answer a target question. Exhibits may include pictures, collages, dioramas, charts and tables, quotes, music, annotated maps, replicas of art, artifacts, primary source documents, time lines, or audiovisual displays. *History Alive!* specifies particular roles for each person in a group and gives criteria for evaluation of the project. Note: The Smithsonian Institute publishes a resource book of four hundred free or inexpensive items available from various museums and organizations, such as posters, slides, and video and audio tapes (see the bibliography).

Classroom Simulations for History

These activities are well-structured and highly motivating. Students participate in an imaginary situation that calls for them to work in groups, to earn points for their group by showing mastery of certain facts, to face a challenge, to make group decisions and act on them, then to evaluate how effective their decisions are. Along with the use of cooperative group skills and higher-order thinking skills, the educational simulations involve students in a good deal of writing on their subject. There are many educational simulations available through various publishers, covering English, social studies, mathematics, and science, ranging in level from elementary through high school. The simulations can take as little as two hours, or as many as forty. Following are descriptions of a few history simulations from Interact (see the bibliography).

Twentieth-Century Activators

In this series of lessons, which range from one to two class periods, students actively experience historical events. In the activity focusing on a Depression-era soup kitchen, students play the roles of hungry, unemployed workers, a preacher, or soup kitchen staff. The hungry clients are made to wait in line then listen to a sermon before being fed soup and scraps of bread (see figures 3-4 and 3-5). The Kent State tragedy of 1970 is reenacted in a similar activity, which students can do outdoors or in a large indoor space. Students take on the roles of taunting, rock-throwing student demonstrators and nervous members of the National Guard. You can simulate rifle shots with a snare drum (see figures 3-6 and 3-7). Other activators include the incarceration of Japanese Americans in 1942, the Holocaust at Auschwitz in 1944, and the Montgomery bus boycott in 1955.

Chapter 3

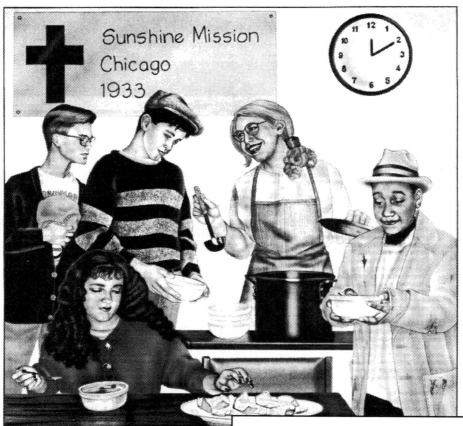

Figure 3-4. Students simulate Depression-era soup kitchen

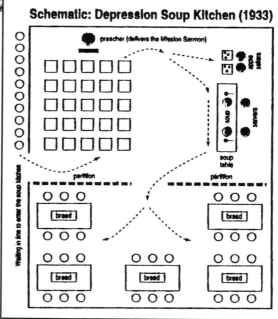

Figure 3-5. Schematic for Depression-era soup kitchen

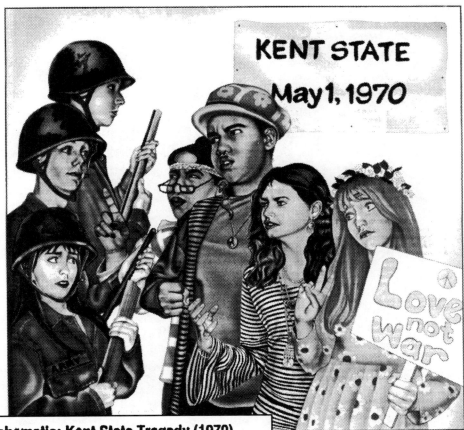

Figure 3-6. Students simulate Kent State tragedy

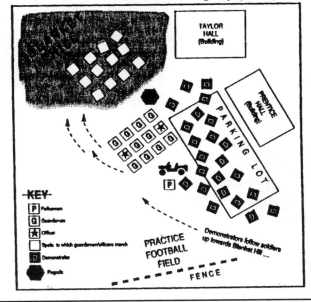

Figure 3-7. Schematic for Kent State tragedy

Trials in World and U.S. History

These activities, three to five periods in duration, reenact the trials of such individuals as Socrates, Joan of Arc, Galileo, and Louis XVI for world history, and Anne Hutchinson, John Brown, Andrew Johnson, John Scopes, and Lt. William Calley for U.S. history. Students play roles of key figures, develop public speaking skills, and debate moral and legal issues using higher-order thinking skills and a range of various intelligences, including the kinesthetic.

Civil War

In this more elaborate simulation that can last from five to thirty class hours, depending on your choice of options, students take on identities and responsibilities of either "Yanks" or "Rebs" and confront one another in simulated combat based on their acquired knowledge. They progress through five stages of the war, experiencing the photography, music, and painting of the time as well as becoming familiar with the economics, logistics, and battles. They express their understanding in letters and journal entries. After an impressive debriefing experience, they take a post-test to demonstrate their increased competencies.

Geography and Economics

"What countries border Iran?"

"Is the country west of Thailand called *Myanmar* or *Burma*?"

Critics of U.S. education often complain that our young people don't know the basics of political geography. In many cases it may be true. A much greater emphasis seems to be placed on geography in European, Asian, Latin American, and African schools than in U.S. schools. Keeping up with basic political geography is especially challenging because borders keep changing. It is possible, though, to liven the teaching of geography by using physical and hands-on activities, including educational simulations.

Map Activities for Geography

I've had good results teaching the locations of countries in each continent by using jigsaw puzzle maps of each continent, with a *separate piece for each country.* (It isn't especially helpful to use the cheaper world map puzzles that are cut into random pieces.) You can buy commercially produced map puzzles or make your own.

Commercially Produced Puzzle Maps

Map puzzles of all the continents are available from Montessori Manipulative Materials: Village Faire for Educators (see bibliography) and other suppliers of Montessori materials. Made of plywood, these maps are large, colorful, and durable, cut out along the lines of the national borders. A small knob for lifting the puzzle piece is attached to each nation's capital. These puzzles' durability is their major advantage. Another advantage is that students can trace individual countries from these puzzle pieces onto paper, making and labeling their own maps of each continent. The puzzles are not generally labeled with the name of the country, so you can write the country name on the back of each piece (and change it if necessary). The disadvantages of commercially produced puzzle maps are that they're expensive, it's hard to replace lost pieces, and if political events change national borders, the map becomes obsolete.

Homemade Map Puzzles

It's less expensive and more conducive to learning to have students make a set of jigsaw puzzle maps themselves. You need two identical large, fairly simplified, double-laminated maps of each continent, clearly showing national borders and capitals. One serves as a reference; the other is cut into jigsaw pieces. The tools for puzzle making are several pairs of good, precise scissors, including a few tiny manicure scissors.

At the beginning of the project, divide the class into six groups, each covering one of the following areas:

    North and Central America
    South America

Europe

Asia

Africa

Australia, Oceania, and Antarctica

Next, give each group the maps you've assigned them. Have the group members cut out the countries from one map *very carefully* along national border lines to form jigsaw puzzle pieces. Island nations such as the Philippines and Indonesia may be cut out as single pieces, surrounded by portions of ocean.

Each group practices putting together the pieces to re-form its continents. When students gain skill with their own puzzles, no longer needing to look at the reference map, they can practice with other continents. Groups can establish speed records in assembling various continents. Some, obviously, are more demanding than others.

People Maps

This activity is a whole-body follow-up to the jigsaw puzzle maps. Choose a continent on which you want the class to focus, and follow these instructions.

1. For each student, make a large card with the name of one or more contiguous countries on the target continent, so all the countries are represented.

2. Provide a large space in which students can sit down.

3. Each student receives a card, face down.

4. At your signal, students turn over the cards and try to arrange themselves in proper places as if they were on a map. As soon as they arrange themselves, they sit and hold their cards over their heads so you or another judge can see how accurately they've arranged themselves. They can try to beat their own speed records for each continent.

Classroom Simulations for Geography and Economics

To learn the cultural and economic aspects of geography, several whole-class simulation activities are available commercially. Following are descriptions of a few geography simulations from Interact, which are listed in the bibliography.

Sanga

This activity, geared toward grades 6 through 9, takes about five hours. After receiving some background information, students take on roles as family members in a village of the Dogon culture in Mali. Each family has certain resources to barter for goods needed. In the highly structured Dogon barter process, disagreements may come up and must be resolved by the wise old healer of the village. Students' success in bartering is assessed, and they finish by evaluating the experience and making cross-cultural comparisons between American and Dogon customs.

Boxcars

This activity is designed for grades 5 through 8 and is estimated to take four hours. Groups of students form shipping companies to move goods by train through western Europe, buying and selling commodities. To trade successfully, they must learn the imports, exports, and profit potentials of the various commodities in each country. The winners are the companies whose profits are highest, because this financial success indicates a more thorough understanding of the economic geography of the area.

Pacific Rim

This activity is appropriate for grades 5 through 8 and takes twenty or more hours. Teams of students gather facts and create projects that relate to some aspect of their countries, then share the projects with the rest of the class. Next, they undertake a race from New Zealand to Japan in imaginary ships. By responding well to certain factual challenges and meeting various twists of fate, they plot their progress on a route outlined on a large map, receiving visas from each country they pass. In their summation, students compare and contrast the countries and discuss implications for immigrants, travelers, and businesspeople. In a final festival, the class celebrates with local foods, kite contests, and other authentic experiences.

Sample Script: Imaginary Journey in History

Escape from Srebrenica

Come with me in your imagination to a place where the world learned a bitter lesson. We're going to Bosnia, a small country in what used to be Yugoslavia in eastern Europe.

Close your eyes and imagine that you're a seventeen-year-old Muslim boy in the eastern Bosnian city of Srebrenica in early July 1995. You're gnawing on a piece of dry bread and your feet are sore and tired. You came here like 40,000 other people because the Bosnian Serb army took over your town, killing hundreds of people, including your father. Your mother hid you in a secret part of the cellar just before she and your sisters were taken away in buses. "Go to Srebrenica as soon as you can," she said. "The U.N. has sent peacekeepers to make it a safe place for Muslims. If Allah is willing, we'll meet you there."

As you wander through the streets looking for your family, you hear people talking. "They said we had to leave our bakery because we're Muslims," says an old woman. "They say they're getting revenge because the Turks were Muslims and they killed a lot of Serbs when they ruled our country. That was long ago, and besides, we're not Turks. We speak the same language as the Serbs. We even look like them, may Allah forgive us."

"We all lived together in peace until Yugoslavia broke up," says a man on crutches. "In my town I had neighbors who were Serbs. My little boy's best friend was a Croat. What does it matter if there were some Croats who helped the fascists? That was more than fifty years ago."

"When Tito's communists were in power, anybody who stirred up trouble was arrested. Now we're supposed to be free and we get killed by our neighbors," the old woman replies.

The old man growls, "Karadzic knew he couldn't get elected in Bosnia so he stirred up the Serbs to hate the Muslims and the Croats. He's acting like Hitler."

There are rumors that the Serb army has surrounded Srebrenica and is about to take over the city. "Why doesn't the U.N. do something?" an old man asks.

"The U.N. is weak," another sneers. "The Bosnian Serb soldiers know they can bully the U.N. peacekeepers. And the rest of the world doesn't want to believe that such things are really happening in Bosnia. They don't want to be bothered with us."

Night falls; you huddle in a doorway. In the chilly dawn you're startled awake by the roar of engines. The Bosnian Serb army has invaded the town. The streets are full of soldiers carrying automatic rifles. Hurrying out to the street, you hear someone say, "We're going to Tuzla; it's safe there."

"No," says another. "You have to walk for days across land that's controlled by Serbs. They'll hunt you down like rabbits."

With hundreds of other Muslims, you crowd into the military camp of the U.N. peacekeepers, but the Serbs go right in after you. The Bosnian Serb commander thunders into town with a convoy of buses and trucks, followed by a video crew. You see him smile for the cameras, giving a candy bar to a child and saying, "Don't be afraid. No one will harm you." You hide and watch the other Muslims lining up to get in the buses for evacuation.

The Serb soldiers begin taking the men and boys away somewhere as the U.N. peacekeepers stand by helplessly. You see a man carrying a one-year-old baby, the only surviving member of his family. Desperately he begs a nurse, a volunteer from Germany, to take the baby and keep it safe. She writes his name, hoping that he'll survive to be reunited with his child some day. With tears in her eyes she takes the baby as the soldiers hurry the father off. Your stomach turns in knots as you hear the women and children wail and scream as their husbands, fathers, and brothers are taken away. The soldiers push the women and children into the buses that roar off, one after another.

Running to the other side of town, you see hundreds of people trying to get away to Tuzla. In the confusion, you find

Chapter 3

your way to an abandoned warehouse and hide under a pile of trash until dark, as the soldiers hunt down the refugees. After sunset you set off, managing to elude the spotlights. All night you travel, running and walking. At daybreak you sleep under a clump of bushes. After the second night, you and several others stumble into an ambush. Surrounded by soldiers, there's nothing to do but surrender.

All the men and boys from your group are loaded onto trucks that bump along the roads for hours. You and the others comfort one another as well as you can. A few men have a little bit of bread to eat. One of them shares his supply with you and several others. It's the first food you've had in two days. You choke it down in spite of your dry throat and churning stomach. "Try to keep up your strength," he says. "You're young. Maybe you can escape and tell the world what's going on here."

When the truck stops, the soldiers take out about five men and lock the door. You hear shots. You feel like vomiting, but you can't. You grit your teeth as they take five more men. You hear more shots. Finally, it's your turn. The soldiers yank you and several others out. In the moonlight, you can see the field covered with bodies. "Lie down!" barks a soldier with an AK-47. You stumble and begin to fall as you hear the rifle shots. You feel a pain in your right arm. A man falls near you, wounded and screaming.

You hear the heavy boots of soldiers coming to check the bodies. One almost steps on you, but he goes on and shoots several times into the screaming man, the man who shared his bread with you. Your arm hurts so much that you'd like the soldier to kill you too. You almost call to him, but instead you decide to hang on, to try to get out and tell the horrible story. Sick from the stench of blood, you lie as still as the death around you.

Clouds cover the full moon just as you hear the bulldozers coming. You drag yourself to the other end of the field, where the bodies have already been covered with dirt. You burrow unseen into the loose soil. A couple of soldiers stroll past, smoking cigarettes and sharing a bottle. You hear one of them say, "That was a good hunt. There were a lot of rabbits here."

You lie there in agony, drifting in and out of consciousness. Awakening, you hear the trucks roar off. The bulldozers are quiet. In the moonlight you see some hills about half a kilometer away. You stagger through the darkness into a canyon and find a sheep trough, where you drink the stagnant water gratefully and wash the throbbing gashes where the bullets went through your flesh. You crawl into a thicket and sink into exhaustion until the pain of your arm awakens you. It's full daylight. You risk another trip to the trough, where you drink again. You can barely crawl back to the thicket before you lose consciousness. That night your head is throbbing as you stagger farther into the hills. At dawn a drenching rain begins to fall. An old shed stands next to a tree. You collapse in a corner where the roof doesn't leak.

You're tossing with nightmares—automatic rifle fire, screams, bodies crumpling, the roar of the bulldozers—dogs barking! You open your eyes, leaping to your feet. Two sheep dogs are running toward the shed, growling. "Come back here, you dogs!" an old voice shouts. The dogs step back but stand their ground, growling. An old woman hobbles into the shed.

"Holy Sofia, someone survived! You dogs get out of here! Sit down, young man. You need some help. My little grandson and I will hide you until we can get you to safety. We Serbs are not all butchers like those soldiers."

Four weeks later, you're in Tuzla. A U.S. official is there, talking to survivors from Srebrenica. You add your story to the rest. There's enough evidence to prove that the Bosnian Serb army has committed war crimes. Before long, NATO planes are bombing Bosnian Serb military facilities. The army from neighboring Croatia has pushed the Serbs out of its territory and weakened them further. Several Bosnian Serb leaders have been indicted as war criminals.

At last peace talks begin. Will Serbs, Croats, and Muslims ever be able to live together peacefully? Will your nightmares ever stop? . . .

Let your imagination leave Bosnia now and come back to our classroom. Quietly write a paragraph, draw a picture, or discuss with a friend your experience in escaping from Srebrenica.

4 Mathematics and the Natural Sciences

Mathematics

A New Challenge in the Math Class

As a math teacher, you've probably read the standards of the National Council of Teachers of Mathematics and other publications that advocate using a wider range of teaching techniques. In previous years, math courses, especially in high school, often served as a filter, eliminating students who weren't analytically gifted. Math teachers were expected to be good mathematicians, not necessarily inclusive educators. Now economic necessity requires that we do a better job with a wider clientele. If we want to compete in the international economy, we need a workforce highly literate in mathematics and science. Moreover, by neglecting the mathematical development of economically disadvantaged students, we not only prolong the cycle of poverty, we worsen it. It is becoming widely accepted that our schools need to adopt practices that make math accessible to virtually all students. That means teaching more effectively to a wide range of students from the beginning through middle and high school, a heavy challenge for math teachers.

From Concrete to Abstract

Kinesthetic activities can serve as one key to this challenge. Math is abstract, of course, but it's drawn from concrete phenomena. Introducing a mathematical concept through a concrete experience, with an appropriate passage to abstraction, makes teaching math more rewarding for you and learning it more rewarding for your students. Moreover, kinesthetic activities generally involve other intelligences as well, especially spatial, interpersonal, and rhythmic.

In some regions, mathematicians and teachers are working on restructuring the whole math program to heighten its effectiveness. Even if your school isn't among these schools, however, there are kinesthetic techniques you can insert into your regular curriculum to make math more accessible to more students. First I describe an ambitious, wide-ranging program called the Algebra Project, which is an excellent example of passage from concrete to abstract. Then I suggest several additional activities that can be used without a complete restructuring of curriculum.

Making Big Changes: The Algebra Project

Based in Cambridge, Massachusetts, the Algebra Project has been used to teach algebra successfully to disadvantaged youngsters since the early 1980s. Originated by Robert Moses, a mathematician, educator, and social activist, this program has worked well for seventh and eighth grade students in such diverse settings as northern inner city schools and southern rural poor communities. Its purpose is to prepare students to take advanced math and science courses in high school, giving them the skills they need to succeed in our technological society. The program is summarized in a *Smithsonian* article entitled "If a = math and b = magic" (Watson 1996), and detailed information about it is available from the Algebra Project headquarters (see bibliography).

For each new algebraic concept, students move through five steps.

1. They experience a physical event.
2. They draw pictures or make graphic representations of the event.

3. They write about the event in everyday language.
4. They translate the event into structured mathematical language.
5. They use abstract symbols to represent the event.

Following is an example of an activity used to introduce the concept of algebraic subtraction. Students walk a straight line for several blocks in one direction from their school. They jot down notes and make rough sketches about the path. They return to their school and walk a straight line for several blocks in the opposite direction, taking notes and making sketches. When they return, they create pictures, diagrams, or three-dimensional models of the paths. In cooperative groups, they write about their walk in everyday language, then translate the concepts into mathematical terms. They may designate the school as zero and give each street corner a number. The first block eastward may be +1, the second +2, and so on. The first block westward may be -1, the second -2, and so forth. The students will be able to use equations to express various locations. Later they may use various starting points and calculate the number of blocks in between, using the appropriate integers.

Through their participation in this project, students experience the algebraic fact that numbers mean not only "How many?" but also "In what direction?" As students explain concepts to one another, they learn to communicate with numbers. What used to be abstract symbols become as comprehensible as words. A large percentage of Algebra Project students have been able to skip the usual ninth-grade algebra and go directly into more advanced courses.

The five-step approach of the Algebra Project, as you might have noticed in this example, is exceptionally suited to integrating several intelligences: bodily-kinesthetic, visual-spatial, interpersonal, verbal, and mathematical-logical. Another part of the program involves the use of African drumming patterns to teach ratio and proportion, a method that activates the musical-rhythmic intelligence.

Chapter 4

Starting Small: The Art of the Possible

As we've mentioned, the Algebra Project is an example of a major restructuring of a middle school math program. Although you may not be in a position to restructure, you can add a bodily-kinesthetic intelligence aspect to your teaching. You may be using some of the following ideas already, but others may be new to you.

Computer Math Games That Incorporate Hand-Eye Coordination

The *Math Blaster* and *Alge-Blaster* programs from Davidson and Associates are good examples of these programs. Both are available Windows and Macintosh systems.

Geometric Drawings and Whole-Body Geometric Shapes

Geometry teachers show their students how to use a compass, protractor, and straight edge. This long-standing practice is an excellent kinesthetic activity. In a whole-body variation of this exercise, students manipulate long pieces of elastic or rope to form geometric shapes. A detailed description of this activity appears in unit 7 of the Glencoe/McGraw-Hill series *Interactive Mathematics*.

Acting Out Word Problems

When students find themselves stumped by a word problem, they can often get help by acting it out. If each member of a group represents an element of the problem, all members think more closely about the meaning of the words. A slightly more sophisticated variation is to use the kinesthetic imagination to act out the problem without moving. For example, your students may be trying to solve this problem: "Light travels at a speed of 297,600 km/second. If the circumference of Earth at the equator is about 39,800 km, about how many times could light travel around the equator in one second?" You might give the following suggestion:

Optional Script

In your kinesthetic imagination, put on your brand-new light-speed tennis shoes and get on your mark at the intersection of the prime meridian and the equator. Feel yourself ready to go, at the speed of light, all the way around Earth, following the equator. On your mark, get set, GO! You zoom around Earth at a speed of 297,600 kilometers per second. Remember that the distance around is about 39,800 kilometers. You keep zooming for one second. Each time you pass the starting line, your light-speed lap counter tells how many times you've circled Earth. At the end of the second, you stop. Uh-oh! Your lap counter has malfunctioned, but not to worry; you have another way of figuring it out. Each time you went around, it was a piece of 297,600 kilometers that was 39,800 kilometers long. How many of those pieces were there? What do you do to find out?

Manipulative Math Materials

Many teachers used to think that manipulatives were only for primary grades, but many work well for introducing certain middle school and high school math concepts. Some newer basal math textbook series include manipulatives up to the eighth grade level. Traditional hands-on Montessori materials concretize such concepts as the cube of a binomial or trinomial, the square root, and the cube root.

Manipulatives for Prealgebra and Algebra

The book *Get It Together* (1989) by Tim Erickson is full of highly motivating problems for cooperative groups. Many of them use manipulatives. One, "Four Kids with Beans," designed for prealgebra classes, demonstrates the concepts of variables and sums of unknowns. Students solve simultaneous equations using two kinds of manipulatives, which may be paper clips, dry pasta shells, or any other small, inexpensive items. In one example, four kids have twenty-five beans among them. Kris and Moira together have nine. Erin and Jay together have sixteen. Students place manipulatives next to labels with the kids' names and with a few more hints, they figure out how many beans each kid has.

"Wodjah and Company," a more demanding game in the same book, is good for high school algebra students. Students can use manipulatives to solve its more complex word problems in such areas as probability and physics.

Shooting Mathematical Baskets

After each student in a group has taken a certain number of shots at the basket, students look at their scores and derive percentages and probability conclusions. Students can do this activity outdoors, in a gym, or with a bean bag and trash can in the classroom.

Designing a House

Give students figures for maximum expenditures and maximum square footage, and have them design their ideal houses, including dimensions. This challenge can be as simple or as sophisticated as you wish.

Mathematical Celebrity Party

Each student has taped to her back a sign with a mathematical term, a formula, a key concept, or any other simple item you want to emphasize. Students try to guess their celebrity identities by asking yes-no questions. Students can do this activity individually in front of the class, in small groups, or as a whole class with students mingling and asking questions.

Math Simulation Games

In these imaginative and well-structured games, the class is divided into small groups to solve problems. For example, in the game *Math Quest* produced by Interact (see bibliography), students use problem-solving strategies to progress through several levels, becoming Calculatricians, Geomagicians who match wits with Sir Cumference, Newtonians who evade the frightful Guzinda, and finally Einsteinians, who, armed with the theory of relativity, are capable of outwitting the dreaded Teacherasaurus.

Additional sources of ideas for active math learning can be found in the bibliography.

Natural Sciences

You have undoubtedly used plenty of hands-on activities with your science students, such as lab demonstrations, experiments, and science fair projects. This section's purpose, then, is to suggest other, less traditional types of kinesthetic techniques for the science curriculum. I begin with a selection of kinesthetic activities ranging from simple to more complex. A later section features information about Richard Shope's work in a NASA educational outreach program. The program includes a sophisticated use of whole-body activities as metaphors to help students understand abstract, unfamiliar ideas. The sample script at the end of the chapter allows students to let their kinesthetic imaginations transport them into an atom.

Starters

The following two activities, versions of those used in other chapters, function well as starters to learn new concepts or as reinforcement of concepts already introduced.

Imaginary Journeys in Science

Students use their kinesthetic imaginations to journey into states of being that would be otherwise inaccessible. See the sample script "Journey into an Atom" at the end of this chapter.

Scientific Celebrity Party

Each student has taped to his back a sign with a scientific term, a formula, an element of the periodic table, or any other item you want to emphasize. Students try to guess their celebrity identities by asking yes-no questions. Students can do this activity individually in front of the class, in small groups, or as a whole class, with students mingling and asking questions.

Scientific Skits

Students perform skits or pantomimes dramatizing the formation of chemical compounds, the circulation of blood, the movement of tectonic plates, or any of a number of scientific phenomena.

Tech Terms Rondo Rap

This activity, which Gail Herman teaches in her seminars, can help students learn all kinds of content. For instance, you can use this activity to teach middle school students the elements of the periodic table. The pattern itself is the simple rondo form used in classical music: A B, A C, A D, and so on. Once students have the idea, they can make up a rhyming couplet for each element, accompanied by clapping, snapping, tapping, or dancing. Following is an example:

A. Out on the court, shootin' around,

   Periodic table comin' down.

B. First dude steps up, what's his name?

   Hydrogen, hydrogen, he gets in the game.

A. Out on the court, shootin' around,

   Periodic table comin' down.

C. Second dude shoots one, what's his line?

   Helium, helium, doin' fine.

A. Out on the court, shootin' around,

   Periodic table comin' down.

Science Museum

Students can set up their own hands-on interactive museum using suggestions from the book *Shapes, Loops, and Images* by Janet Jagoda and her group. The book tells how to set up exhibits using single mirrors to demonstrate lines of symmetry and multiple mirrors for patterns of geometry.

Students can make giant pole puzzles to learn spatial relationships and topology, and tessellations to find, analyze, and relate patterns. Having experienced this kind of museum-making, students can go on to design and build original exhibits.

Science Simulations

In these imaginative whole-class activities, students learn about subject matter while developing cooperative and higher-order thinking skills. Following are descriptions of two simulations from Interact (see the bibliography).

Balance

Geared toward grades 9 through 12, this activity is estimated to take sixteen to thirty-five hours. In the first part of this two-part environmental simulation, students take on the roles of animals, American Indians, and settlers in a capsule simulation of the ecological effect of subduing the wilderness. In the second part, the class is divided into families who live in growing cities that have serious ecological problems. Students stretch their abilities to balance short-range, personal satisfaction with long-range ecological health.

Clone

Designed for grades 8 through 12 and estimated to last six to ten hours, this simulation is of a congressional hearing on genetic engineering. Students take on the roles of senators, witnesses, attorneys, biologists, and two cloned beings, Eugenia and Eugene. Students present and hear testimony, conduct debates, then write a culminating paragraph or theme on what it is to be human.

Pluto Express Educational Outreach

The National Aeronautics and Space Administration (NASA) conducts educational outreach programs in connection with each of its space exploration projects. One project in the planning stage is the spacecraft to Pluto, scheduled to be launched in the early years of the twenty-first century. NASA's Pluto Express Educational Outreach materials are free to schools (see bibliography). They contain a wealth of ideas for experiential science learning developed by Richard Shope, a highly creative educator who draws on his background as a professional mime artist. The kinesthetic activities, some of which Shope discussed with me during conversations in 1995 and 1996, demonstrate concepts as simple as interplanetary distances and as highly abstract as the fourth state of matter (plasma) and its relation to the solar wind and the earth's magnetosphere. I've summarized two of the activities here. You can contact the Pluto Express Educational Outreach for the additional materials.

Interplanetary Distances

Scientists use a convenient unit to measure distances between the planets of our solar system, the astronomical unit, equivalent to the average distance between the Sun and Earth (about 93 million miles). This activity gives a kinesthetic sense of the kinds of distances in our solar system.

Interplanetary Distance Chart
(average distances from sun in astronomical units [a.u.])

Sun	0.0
Mercury	0.4
Venus	0.7
Earth	1.0
Mars	1.5
Asteroid belt	2.8–3.0
Jupiter	5.2
Saturn	9.5
Uranus	19.2
Neptune	30.0
Pluto	39.0

Students work in teams of eleven to fifteen each. Each team chooses a way of representing an astronomical unit (such as a team member with arms outstretched). The teams go to a large space such as an athletic field or a nearby park. Their task is to make a scale model of the relative distances between the planets, with each team member acting as one of the objects in the solar system. Several students can serve as asteroids.

Once the planets are in place, you can set the solar system in motion. Each orbit is slightly elliptical, except for Pluto's, which is more eccentric. Pluto is tilted about 170 degrees out of the elliptical plane of the planets. As students orbit counter-clockwise, they may find it a challenge to avoid drifting in toward the Sun. If you wish, on their second time around, students can mark their orbits with string.

In an extension of the activity, students consider the relative distances beyond the solar system. If students have judged the relative distance of Pluto from the Sun as across the athletic field, how far is our nearest cluster of stars, Alpha Centauri?

Solar Wind, Plasma, Magnetospheres, and Auroras

This activity is one of Richard Shope's highly creative and complex activities, and I describe it here to give you a flavor of what can be done kinesthetically to make abstract scientific concepts understandable to a wide range of students. If you decide to try this one with your students, I suggest you read the instructions ahead of time. Keep the pace lively, the drama intense, and be willing to "ham it up"—get into the motion with students as they dramatize these phenomena. The purpose of this activity is for students to experience a physical metaphor of several abstract, interrelated concepts:

the dynamic activity of the Sun

the fourth state of matter: plasma

the solar wind and its interaction with Earth's magnetosphere

the production of the auroras

Chapter 4

Background Information

Introduce this background information as a quick lecture, then follow with the physical activity to help students internalize the concepts.

Magnetospheres

We can't see them or feel them, but magnetic fields are all around us and we use them every time we start an electric motor, navigate with a compass, or watch a video. We know a good deal about how magnetism works in everyday life, but we're still learning about the magnetic fields, called *magnetospheres*, that exist around certain planets, including Earth.

It was only in 1958 that scientists began to understand the importance of Earth's magnetosphere. During that year the Geiger counters aboard *Explorer I*, the first American satellite in space, went crazy at certain altitudes. James Van Allen and other scientists later explained the problem by identifying a doughnut-shaped belt of energetic particles that were trapped by the magnetosphere. This belt was named after Van Allen. Later space flights mapped Earth's magnetosphere quite accurately.

Scientists have many different opinions about what magnetospheres are and how they occur. One theory is that Earth's core of hot nickel and iron moves as Earth rotates, acting as a magnetic dynamo. Other planets, however, are composed of different elements. Some have strong magnetospheres and others have virtually none at all.

Plasma, the Fourth State of Matter

Most of us learned in elementary school that there are three states of matter: solid, liquid, and gas. We were taught that matter changes among these three states because of temperature. During the last fifty years, however, scientists have been learning more about a fourth state of matter called *plasma*, a fully ionized gas (which is, of course, different from the plasma that is part of our blood). They have estimated that more than 99 percent of the matter in the universe exists as plasma.

If so much of the universe is in plasma form, why did it take us so long to learn about it? It's mainly because matter usually enters the plasma state only under conditions of extremely high temperature and powerful electromagnetic waves. On Earth, these conditions don't exist naturally and are generally limited to laboratories doing research in nuclear fusion. There are a few exceptions, though. Everyday examples of the use of plasma are fluorescent or neon lights. The special gases inside the tubes are able to ionize easily when exposed to an electromagnetic field. The gases release energy in the form of light as they ionize.

Solar Wind

Most of the sun's matter is in the plasma state, so it behaves differently than it would as a solid, liquid, or gas. This plasma is hot stuff, at temperatures from nine thousand to twenty million degrees Kelvin. It moves supersonically in wave patterns, it gives off radiant energy, and it is highly charged electrically. As the Sun rotates on its axis, streams of plasma are thrown off spirally at enormous speeds. These plasma streams traveling through space are called the *solar wind* (see figure 4-1).

Figure 4-1. Spiral path of solar wind

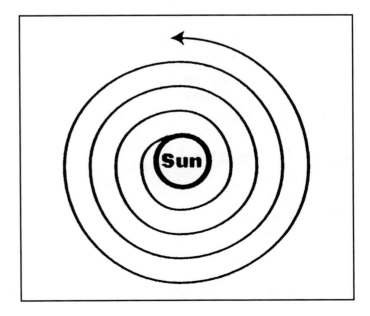

There's plenty of room for the streams of plasma that comprise the solar wind to spread out in interplanetary space so they have low density but high energy. When these huge low-density sheets of plasma hit planetary magnetospheres, they don't collide with the magnetospheres. Instead, they act like water does in a swift stream when it comes to a boulder: they part and go around the obstacle. This parting is called *bow shock* (as in the bow of a ship).

A Universe of Plasma

Scientists generally assume that the other stars in the universe are similar to our sun in that they have extremely high temperatures and intense electromagnetic energy. Scientists surmise that the vast majority of stellar matter is in the plasma state and that high-speed, low-density plasma radiates throughout interstellar space. For that reason, scientists believe that a vast percentage of the matter in the universe is in the form of plasma rather than in a solid, liquid, or gaseous state.

Activity

Before beginning this activity, you might want to choose at least four students who enjoy being spontaneous and in the spotlight for a special role at the end: the "dancing light show" of the auroras. Without giving away your plan to the rest of the group, assign at least two students to be parts of the Sun's photosphere (later becoming solar wind particles) and at least two others to be part of Earth's magnetosphere.

Optional Script

You've been listening to a lot of abstract information, so let's make it more concrete. That way it's likely to make more sense and become part of you.

We all know that the Sun is more than just a big smiling circle in the sky. It's always shining—day and night! Yes, of course, we go to sleep at night, but the Sun still shines on the other side of Earth. The center of the Sun is tremendously powerful, terribly hot, and always, always active. Is there anybody who would like to be this powerful, hot, active center of the Sun? Choose between one and five students. Have them get up and start moving in some way that represents the intense energy of the Sun. Move with them and encourage them to make up their own motions. Once they're started, you can move away from the center. If they stop moving, remind them lightheartedly that there is no rest for the Sun. They keep going while you set up the next part of the picture.

So far we have the center of the Sun. Now we need some volunteers to be the Sun's photosphere, the visible light region of the Sun that we can see in the sky. Select three to seven or more students to represent the photosphere, including at least two of the capable limelight-seekers you identified earlier. Arrange them around the Sun as you explain the following.

Remember, most of the Sun's matter is in the plasma form. This outer group represents the plasma particles that move out from the Sun all the time. We're creating just one brief snapshot of something that's really happening constantly, night and day, all year round. Okay, outer group, remember that you're plasma particles, which means you're highly charged with energy. Wave your arms to show this energy. But you don't just stay close to the Sun. The center of the Sun is rotating with so much energy that in a minute you plasma particles will go flying off in vast sheets, spiraling through the solar system and going far beyond the distance of the planets. Real plasma sheets move at almost a million miles an hour, but you'll show us in slow motion. These plasma sheets are what we mean by the solar wind. Have the solar wind students move in spiral paths out from the center, waving their arms. Point out that the *Voyager* spacecraft is still detecting solar wind more than one hundred times as far from the Sun as we are on Earth! (That's more than one hundred astronomical units.)

Okay, everyone rest for a moment—even the solar wind and the center of the Sun. Before we have you start moving again, let's put Earth into the system. For some time we've known that the solar wind interacts with Earth's magnetosphere now and then. It can cause electromagnetic storms that affect telecommunications.

More recently, scientists have learned more about how the solar wind behaves when it approaches Earth. Recruit one or more volunteers to stand together and represent Earth. Have at least one of them face the Sun. Then recruit several students to serve as Earth's magnetosphere, including at least two of the spontaneous students you identified earlier. Have them circle a short distance out and around Earth, waving their arms to represent the magnetic field. *What do you think is going to happen when the solar wind approaches Earth? Let's have the solar wind people approach in slow motion.*

At this point, you may want to heighten the drama by stopping the solar wind students just before they reach Earth's magnetosphere. Have students conjecture what may happen, and have students act out any students' conjectures. If any are correct, go on from there; if not, have students re-form just short of the encounter between the solar wind and the magnetosphere. Select a student to represent the bow shock, standing just between the solar wind and the magnetosphere students. *The bow shock isn't actually a physical entity. It's really a shock wave that comes from the solar wind's magnetic force pushing on the magnetosphere's force. It creates a pattern of movement like the bow of a boat when it's going through the water. There isn't a physical collision of particles. The bow shock directs the solar wind around the outside of the magnetosphere to the dark side of Earth. So bow shock person, act like a traffic cop and direct some solar wind people to the right and some to the left as they approach you. In reality, the solar wind would also go up and over, down and below Earth, but for this activity we're restricted by gravity, so our solar wind people will just go to the right and left. And everyone remember that nobody actually bumps into anyone else. The solar wind is directed* around *Earth's magnetosphere.*

As the solar wind goes around Earth, it has two effects. It compresses the magnetosphere on the light side of Earth. The bow shock person and the magnetosphere people on the light side can represent this compression by moving slightly backward toward Earth as the solar wind goes around you. The solar wind also draws the dark side of the magnetosphere into a long, skinny tail. Let's have some of the magnetosphere people form that skinny tail on the dark side of Earth, where it's night time. Include your spontaneous limelight seekers in this tail.

Suddenly, somewhere here on the dark side, some sheets of solar wind particles interact with the magnetosphere and produce dancing light shows called the auroras.

At this point, give a signal to the spontaneous students from the solar wind and the magnetosphere to make up a dance or some funny or dramatic movement that represents the auroras. This is where the *Aha!* experience happens. Students recognize that the whole pattern fits together as a unity and a system: sun, solar wind, plasma, magnetosphere, and auroras (see figure 4-2), and that the elements of the solar system interact in various ways. While the

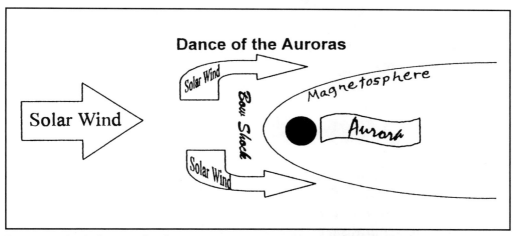

Figure 4-2. Solar wind, plasma, magnetospheres, and auroras

dance is going on, you may want to explain that the auroras are generally seen by people fairly close to the poles. The aurora borealis occurs near the North Pole and is sometimes called the northern lights. The aurora australis is seen near the South Pole.

If students are receptive and time allows, have them repeat the activity in whole or in part, so they can play various roles and others make up their own dancing light shows.

Chapter 4

Follow-up Suggestions

- Draw pictures or diagrams, including labels and captions, to illustrate the following concepts: *magnetosphere, plasma, solar wind, bow shock, aurora borealis, aurora australis.* You may use one drawing to illustrate several concepts. In groups of four, compare your diagrams and write a description of how the Sun gives off solar wind and what happens when the wind come close to Earth.

- Discuss the following questions.

   How do we use magnetic fields in everyday life?

   In what ways is the plasma state of matter different from the solid, liquid, and gaseous states?

   Why is the plasma state of matter so difficult to observe on Earth?

   How do fluorescent and neon lights use the plasma state of matter?

- Construct a three-dimensional model showing the Sun, the solar wind, Earth's magnetosphere, the poles, and the auroras. Research the following questions independently.

   When and how did scientists first begin to realize the full importance of Earth's magnetosphere?

   What does the Van Allen belt have to do with the magnetosphere's importance?

   What instruments are used to explore Earth's magnetosphere?

   How do space scientists learn about magnetospheres of other planets?

   Which planets have magnetospheres?

   Why is it that some planets do not have magnetospheres?

   What might happen to life on Earth if our magnetosphere didn't deflect most of the solar wind?

Sample Script: Imaginary Journey in Science

Journey into an Atom

Sit fairly straight and breathe deeply and comfortably. Close your eyes. Feel the air going in and out of your lungs. Let yourself sense the circulation in your veins and arteries, the workings of your muscles and nerves. Feel how well all the various elements in your body are working together to keep you healthy.

Focus your concentration on your left hand. Now move your attention down to the tip of your left index finger. Keeping your eyes closed, let your mind see what your fingertip looks like. Become deeply aware of the tip of that one finger. Think about the fingernail, the layers of skin, the small precise muscles, the tiny veins and arteries, the little bone that provides the structure. Let your sensory nerves feel the sensations in that fingertip.

Your whole body is made up of tiny cells that work together in marvelous ways. Right now you're going to become one of those cells in your fingertip. Decide for yourself whether you'll be a skin cell, a muscle cell, a red or white blood cell, or perhaps a nerve cell that carries messages from your brain or back to it. Let yourself sense what it's like to be a cell. Around the outside of you is your cell membrane, which is your boundary and window to the rest of the cells. At your center is your nucleus, the command center of the cell. Sense the chemical activity going on in the cell as it takes in nourishment and turns it into energy.

Most cells have a certain amount of water in them, so look around and find a molecule of water. You'll recognize it because it's made of two atoms of hydrogen and one atom of oxygen. Go into that tiny molecule and feel what it's like to be such a simple structure—made up of just three atoms. Feel the connections that hold these atoms together. Feel how the atoms cooperate to make up a molecule of water.

Now make yourself extremely tiny and climb into one of the hydrogen atoms. You feel yourself getting even tinier as you drift into the center of the hydrogen atom, the nucleus. You watch for the outer particle, the electron, spinning around the outside. It doesn't orbit in a regular pattern, like Earth orbits the Sun. As a matter of fact, you're never exactly sure where the electron is;

you can only make a good guess. Now you're the size of the tiny proton in the nucleus of the hydrogen atom. Suddenly the rest of the atom seems enormous as you spin there in the center of it. The electron is somewhere out there, so tiny and far from you. You're amazed at how much empty space there is inside an atom.

Now it's time to see what's even smaller than the proton. You make yourself unimaginably tiny to find out what the proton is made of, and suddenly you enter the world of the vast, wonderful mystery. Scientists, with their sophisticated equipment and their particle accelerators, have tried to find out what's inside the tiny subatomic particles such as electrons, protons, and neutrons. What they've found is a marvelous world of puzzles and contradictions, of probabilities and patterns of energy. There seem to be some elusive entities called quarks that are even tinier than protons, but very little is known about them. Scientists look for clues in the patterns of energy created inside the subatomic particles. Let yourself fly and turn flips and float and dance around in this energy for a while . . . Feel the energy flow through you and feel yourself flowing through the energy. Let yourself sense the connection between this energy and the forces that make up the rest of the cosmos.

Now that you've found a way to visit the inside of an atom, it's time to return home. Make yourself the size of the proton again and spin around in the nucleus of the atom . . . Begin to get bigger, and now you're the size of the atom itself. You see the other hydrogen atom and the oxygen atom that make up the water molecule, and gradually you become the size of the whole molecule. You flow around comfortably inside the cell for a while and gradually grow to the size of the whole cell.

Now you're getting larger, and you're the size of your fingertip. You let your attention expand and you're the size of your whole hand. Your consciousness spreads through your whole body. You feel the air going in and out of your lungs as you breathe. You sense the circulation in your hands and feet, in your arms and legs, your hips, your back and chest, your neck and head, and your face.

Before you open your eyes, let yourself smile and remember what it was like in that world of energy inside an atom . . .

Mathematics and the Natural Sciences

Now slowly open your eyes and look around. Without speaking, look at the people and the things around you and remember that they're made of cells, molecules, atoms, and tiny particles such as protons. Remember that those tiny particles are made up of something that seems to be pure energy. Let yourself feel that energy now, the energy that connects everything in the universe . . . the energy that combines to make mountains and monsters, people and dreams, the energy that dissolves and recombines, so that everything—even the planet—will eventually change into something different.

As you look around, feel yourself growing and changing. Feel the energy that connects you and everything in the universe.

Now, without talking, draw a picture or write a paragraph about what you saw and what you felt on this imaginary journey inside an atom.

5 Study Skills, Self-Management, and Conflict Resolution

Study Skills: The Brain-Body Connection

A great deal of research in the last two decades has confirmed that learning is not a function only of the brain. Even highly abstract academic learning can be enhanced through appropriate physical activity.

Our understanding of the brain took a leap when Nobel Prize winner Roger Sperry demonstrated that the two cerebral hemispheres of the brain tend to be specialized for different functions, almost like two different brains. One side (often the left) tends to specialize in analytic, linear thinking. It is often called the *logic brain*. The other hemisphere (often the right) is sometimes called the *gestalt brain*. It tends to see totalities, to make associations, and to introduce emotion and compassion into thought processes. Each side of the brain is connected to the opposite side of the body. Sounds coming into the right ear, for instance, are processed in the left side of the brain. Movements of the left foot are controlled by the right motor cortex.

The two hemispheres can communicate with each other through a special bundle of nerve fibers called the *corpus callosum*. When this nerve pathway is fully developed, it allows the two hemispheres to work together, resulting in intellectual productivity greater than the sum of what the two brains working individually could produce. Certain physical activities enhance the development of the corpus callosum and other nerve networks. A valuable source of detail on learning and the brain is Carla Hannaford's *Smart Moves*.

Albert Einstein is a good example of a brilliant thinker who enhanced his thinking with activities outside his professional specialty. Throughout his life, he balanced the linear, analytical rigor of the scientist with the holistic, aesthetic relaxation of playing the violin. In the process of moving the bow and fingering the strings, he was coordinating the two sides of the body. This coordination required messages to pass from the right side of the body to the left side of the brain and vice versa, activating and integrating both hemispheres.

Moreover, Einstein was deeply sensitive to messages from his senses and his muscles. He mentioned that his most important insights often came as *feelings in his muscles*, which he later translated into words or mathematical formulas.

We don't all need to be Einsteins or violinists to find activities that enhance the integration of the two hemispheres and other brain functions. This chapter suggests a number of possibilities in addition to internal sensing and self-calming, and the use of the kinesthetic imagination, the two methods described in chapter 1. In this section I describe several activities, then summarize a comprehensive approach called "Brain Gym" developed by Paul Dennison.

Cerebellar Minestrone

How often have you wanted to do four or five things at a time? Perhaps without noticing it, you often do. You probably drive your car, which involves hand, foot, and eye coordination, while watching traffic, while carrying on a conversation, while changing the cassette in the stereo. Doing all these things at once stimulates several areas of your brain, especially the cerebellum and the sensory and motor areas of the cerebral cortex.

You can help your students do the same with this exercise, adapted from a more elaborate one called "Multitracking" in Jean Houston's *The Possible Human* (1982, 72). Aside from its brain-stimulating value, this activity is good for warming up a group that is about to do something challenging, or for reenergizing a class that has sat still for a long time. Feel free to use one or several of the sets of instructions. Be prepared for some giggles.

Optional Script

You probably know already that your body can help your brain work better. We're going to spend a little bit of time waking up some parts of your brain. Please stand next to your desks. Ask students to perform one of these sets; after each set is completed, add an additional set as necessary.

- *Pretend to play the piano with your feet while you snap your fingers. Continue to play and snap while you make big circles with your arms, blink your eyes, and nod your head. Keep doing all those things while you sing, "Row, Row, Row Your Boat" and think about sewing buttons on ice cream.*

- *Do a tap dance, conduct an orchestra with your hands, wiggle your ears, roll your eyes around clockwise, move your head from side to side, sing "Jingle Bells," and remember what you had for lunch yesterday.*

- *Hop on one foot, pretend to play a guitar, wink your left eye, turn your head from side to side, count backward from twenty to zero, and try* not *to picture a polar bear sitting on a cake of ice.*

- *Jog in place, pat the top of your head with your left hand, rub your stomach with your right hand, look up and down, up and down, wink your right eye, sing "The Star-Spangled Banner," and think about a snake riding a unicycle.*

- *Lie on your back, pretend to ride a bicycle with your legs, flap your arms like wings, move your head slowly from side to side, move your eyes in the opposite direction, sing "Happy Birthday," and think about what color the wind is today.*

Your Personal Expert Trainer

Following is a practical application of the kinesthetic imagination to improve a skill. I introduce it in the context of a physical skill, but once students have learned it, they can apply it to intellectual and social skills as well. This activity is an adaptation of one called "Skill Rehearsal with the Master Teacher" from *The Possible Human* by Jean Houston (1982, 177). You need enough space for each student to lie on the floor and practice or simulate a physical skill.

At the beginning, you give students a few minutes to choose a physical skill they would like to improve, one that they can practice or simulate in the space you have available. High dives and triple back flips might be impractical for this activity, but simulating keyboard skills or a tennis serve would be quite feasible. Running can be simulated by jogging in place. You might want to list possible skills on the board. Some suggestions are listed at the end of this activity. Feel free to add other skills that especially interest your students. After choosing an activity, students think of an expert they want for their imaginary teacher.

Have students warm up with two or three sets of activities from "Cerebellar Minestrone" to help awaken the sensory and motor areas of the cerebral cortex. These preliminaries are included in the optional script that follows. It's a good idea to provide some quiet background music for the activity.

Optional Script

You probably know that lots of world-class athletes use their imaginations to help them improve their skills. An NBA player might visualize himself making a perfect three-point shot. He might imagine his muscles moving in ideal coordination and feel

Study Skills, Self-Management, and Conflict Resolution

himself completing the shot. Then he can practice with his physical body, and he usually finds that he performs better than before. Some athletes alternate between mind-practice and physical practice, and they find the combination works better than an equal amount of practice with the physical body alone.

We're going to try something like that. Maybe not all of you are going to be NBA players or Olympic athletes, but you all have some kind of physical skill that you could improve. It may be an athletic skill such as shooting baskets, or it may be a small-muscle activity such as typing faster on your computer keyboard, playing a riff on a guitar, fixing your hair a new way, winning a video game, or dissecting a frog.

I'm going to give you a few minutes to think of a physical skill you'd like to improve, and we'll experiment with using your mind to help you do it. For this experiment, please choose a skill that you can practice or pretend to practice right here. Don't choose something such as skydiving, bronco riding, or high jumping. You can do that on your own, once you've learned this mind-body technique. Give students about three minutes to think of a skill to practice. For those who can't think of anything, assign them to focus on the skill of writing legibly with their nondominant hands.

Now, please think of someone who is an expert at the skill you've chosen. It doesn't have to be someone you know personally. It can be someone who isn't even living any more, such as Babe Ruth to teach you how to bat, or it can be an imaginary character, such as R2D2 to teach you how to program computers. The person you choose will visit your imagination and be your personal expert trainer for this activity. Give students another three minutes to decide on their expert trainer. Those who had trouble choosing a skill may also need help identifying an expert trainer for the skill of writing with their nondominant hands. You might suggest Harry Truman, who could write with either hand. Once students have identified their expert trainers, have them do two or three sets of activities from "Cerebellar Minestrone" to stimulate their brains.

Now, please lie down on the floor, not touching anyone else. Let your body relax as completely as possible. Imagine you're in a boat at the edge of the ocean. You're lying in the sun and drifting comfortably along, feeling the side-to-side rocking of the gentle waves. It's like being in a hammock, only more free. You have a good feeling all over as your boat drifts further out to sea.

Gradually the swells get a little higher and your boat rocks gently up and down. You hear a swishing sound and your boat enters a whirlpool, a gentle whirlpool that takes you around and around very comfortably. You're going down and around, down and around, and you sense that this whirlpool is a friendly place where you don't have to worry about anything. You don't even get very wet. You just whirl gently around and down until your boat comes softly to rest on the bottom of the ocean.

You get out and look up. You can see the blue sky above you through the airy center of the whirlpool. You look behind you and see a door in the ocean floor. You open the door and find a stone staircase. You walk down the stairs and follow the spiral stone staircase down and around some more. There's just enough light to see where you're going. You come to a long hallway lined with sparkling crystals. At the end of the hallway you open another door. It leads into a large, light, airy room: the room of the skill.

There's a friendly person in the room, your personal expert trainer in the skill you want to learn. This expert trainer can teach you much more than you ever knew before. In your mind's eye let yourself see what your expert trainer looks like. What does the person's voice sound like? As your personal trainer demonstrates and you practice the skill, you'll feel as if your muscles are actually performing, even though your physical body is lying still. You'll spend five minutes of clock time with your personal trainer, and it may seem much longer because your brain and nerves and muscles can accomplish a great deal when you are in this special state of mind. You have all the time you need to learn a tremendous amount from your personal trainer. Give students five minutes.

Now it's time to leave. Thank your personal expert trainer and say good-bye. Your expert trainer tells you that you can come back any time and wishes you a happy journey home. As you walk to the door of the room, you see a beautiful green light shining down from the ceiling. You stand under this light for a moment. It's the light that confirms your new knowledge. You feel the skill strengthened, and you can't wait to get home and try it out. You go out of the room and close the door behind you. As you go back through the hallway, you feel the skill growing in you. You walk up the stairway and out the door onto the ocean floor. You close the door and get into your boat. The boat gently lifts itself up into the whirlpool and swirls up and around, up and around, until you get back to the surface of the ocean. The boat rocks and pitches gently toward the shore. You can feel the skill growing in you. You reach the shore, pull the boat up, and step onto the dry sand where you practice the skill again with your kinesthetic imagination.

Now, gently open your eyes and, with your physical body, practice the skill or simulate practicing it. Then practice it with your kinesthetic imagination again. Go back and forth a few times between your physical body and your kinesthetic imagination. Let your body remember all that you learned from your personal expert trainer. Keep in mind that your body will remember this skill so you can practice and continue improving for a long time. Give students some time to practice the skill. Afterward, have them sit down and write, draw pictures, or discuss their visits to their personal expert trainers.

Following are a few skills students might want to work on during this activity: pitching curve balls, hitting home runs with an imaginary bat, shooting baskets, fencing, golfing, typing, drawing, sculpting, throwing pottery, miming, braiding, sewing, knitting, crocheting, performing magic tricks, juggling, writing calligraphy, playing video games, signing, writing with nondominant hand, using chopsticks, and playing a musical instrument.

After students have practiced this technique a few times with you, remind them that they can use it to learn other, nonphysical skills. They can consult an expert trainer to help them write a good essay or to organize their thoughts before a test, as long as they've put in reasonable study effort already. Expert trainers can help them find ways to work out problems with friends, family, or dates. And expert trainers can help them set their own goals and decide what steps they need to take to accomplish the goals.

Chapter 5

Wimpo, Macho, and Mensch Solve a Problem

Students in middle and high school often discourage themselves by plunging unprepared into problem situations. This activity, adapted from George Leonard's work (1983, 247), helps students explore three different ways of approaching a challenge.

To let all students experience this activity, you need enough space for half of the students to walk about six feet in parallel lines. The problem solvers walk from the beginning of this imaginary line toward the solution at the other end, dealing with the problems in between. Demonstrate the process first, then let students try it.

Optional Script

Have you ever noticed that on some days everything seems to be easy for you and on other days things are really hard and nothing seems to go right? It may have to do with the way your body and mind are working together. They can help you feel good about yourself and see the possibilities in your world, or they can get in your way. We're going to experiment with three different ways your body and mind can work, and see which one seems best for solving a problem.

For this demonstration, I'd like a volunteer who will be Problem Solver. I'll be Problem. Choose a reliable volunteer. *Okay, Problem Solver, stand there and I'll stand here (about six feet away). I'll put my arm out just at the level of your shoulders. Your job is to talk in a straight line past me, through my arm. (See figure 5-1.)*

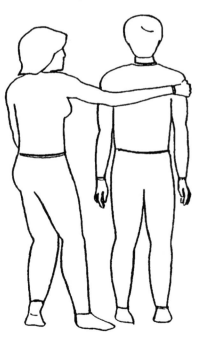

Figure 5-1. Wimpo, Macho, and Mensch solve a problem

Study Skills, Self-Management, and Conflict Resolution

My job is to make it just a bit difficult for you to walk past. Each time you try to walk past me, I'll try to hold you back with the same amount of strength I used the time before. I don't have to try to stop you; I just have to give you the same amount of difficulty each time. Each time you try to walk past me, you're going to be in a different state of mind and body.

The first state of mind and body is the Wimpo mode. Wimpo likes to feel sorry for himself, to feel like a victim. We all get into a Wimpo mood now and then, so Problem Solver, pretend you're Wimpo for a few minutes. Stand with your shoulders hunched over and your head hanging down. Let the corners of your mouth droop. You can say Wimpo things to yourself, such as the following:

- *"Poor little me!"*
- *"Nobody likes me. If they pay any attention to me, it's just because I'm the only one around."*
- *"If I tried, it wouldn't do any good anyway."*
- *"I can't."*

Now, Problem Solver, stay in that Wimpo mood, hunched over, saying lots of Wimpo things, and start walking past me. Keep walking even when you get to my arm and notice how much trouble it is to go past me . . . Ask for reaction.

Now go back to where you started, Problem Solver, and try a different mood, called Macho. Macho thinks he's supposed to be strong all the time. He doesn't show any of his feelings except anger. He takes himself very seriously and he's determined to get his way, no matter what. Just like Wimpo, we all get into a Macho mood now and then, so Problem Solver, pretend to be Macho now. Stand straight, shoulders back, neck muscles tight, arms down by your sides, fists clenched, jaw tight. Walk past me at the same speed you did before. The only change is your mood. See whether it's harder or easier to go past my arm. Notice how you feel while you're doing it . . . What did you notice this time? . . .

Go back to where you started again and we'll try a third way. It's the Mensch mood. Mensch is a Yiddish word for someone who has strength inside, who doesn't have to show it on the outside. If students mention the German meaning of the word, which is somewhat different, congratulate them on knowing it, and return to the Yiddish meaning. *Mensch feels good about the world and helps other people feel good about themselves. A wise person once said, "When a Mensch walks down the street, even the sidewalk feels good." Sometimes you find Mensch characters in stories and movies. One example is Yoda in the Star Wars series. Can you think of any others? . . .*

All of us have a Mensch part of us too, so let yourself get into a Mensch mood now, and we'll all help you. One good way to start feeling like a Mensch is to have a good laugh. Everybody start making silly faces at each other and we'll get a good laugh going . . . Allow a short time for laughs.

Now, Problem Solver, stand with your feet a little apart, breathe deeply and comfortably, let yourself get deeply centered. All of you who are watching, please do the same while you're sitting down, because you'll get a chance to try this in a minute. Close your eyes a moment and think about someone who's a Mensch. It can be someone real or someone from a story. Pretend you're that person. Feel all that good energy flowing through you. You're grounded, relaxed, aware, centered, and deeply energized. Open your eyes. Now, Problem Solver, let your mind and your body walk together in that good energy and walk past me. Notice whether this mood makes it harder or easier to go past me . . . How did it feel? . . .

After the demonstration, have students pair up and take turns being Problem and Problem Solver in each of these three moods. Repeat the instructions to them each time so they get a clear experience of these three different ways of approaching a challenge. They generally find that the Macho mode is more effective than the Wimpo state, and that the Mensch mode is most effective of all. Moreover, the Mensch mode usually has the added advantage of leaving a feeling of harmony between the Problem and the Problem Solver, while the other two modes tend to create a feeling of conflict. Ask for student reactions. Remind them that they can choose to approach any challenge in the Mensch mode, and it's likely to be easier and more pleasant.

Cross-Sensing

Anthropologists say that certain groups of Aborigines routinely talk of having twenty senses or more. They sometimes pity us in "civilization" with our paltry five senses. A highly developed sensorium is a necessity for survival in a harsh environment. Although we and our students may not face the conditions of the outback, we can enhance our sensory perception and our creativity by using an Aboriginal technique, sometimes called *cross-sensing*. This activity is an adaptation of one called *Synesthesia* in Jean Houston's *The Possible Human* (1982, 47). Choose some music that is evocative but somewhat unfamiliar to students. *The Moldau* by Smetana is a selection that often works well. You may want to have art materials available for students to use afterward to express their experience. If it is feasible, have students lie on a reasonably comfortable floor. If not, have them sit and put their heads down on their desks or close their eyes.

Optional Script

You may have heard of people who can get ideas in lots of different ways, not just by thinking in words. Albert Einstein is an example. He said that many of his most important insights came as feelings in his muscles or as visual images. Once he was fully aware of those visual or muscular ideas, he could translate them into words or mathematical formulas. Sometimes this kind of crossover is called cross-sensing.

This activity is meant to give you an experience of cross-sensing. I'm going to play some music, and I'd like you to listen not only with your ears, but with all your senses and your whole body.

Let yourself be as relaxed as possible. Keep your eyes closed. As I play the music, let it flow over you, through you, and around you. Let it become part of you. Let yourself "see" the sound. You may feel as though you're moving with the music, even though your body is actually still. You may sense some fragrances or flavors or textures in the music. Do you notice any change in temperature in the music? Does it seem dark in some places and light in others? Let all these sensations flow through you as you listen with your whole body.

After playing the music, give students some time to savor the experience quietly. Then ask them to write, draw, dance, or discuss with a partner what they felt while the music was playing.

Brain Gym

This program, honored in 1990 by the National Educational Foundation as one of the most effective technologies for education, has been used by people of all ages to enhance learning. A series of simple, nonstrenuous movements presented in stressfree language are done for a few minutes at a time on a regular basis. Originally developed in the 1970s by Paul Dennison of the Educational Kinesiology Foundation, the program is fully outlined in Dennison's many books (1985, 1986, 1994) and is also highlighted in Carla Hannaford's video and recent book (1993, 1995). Here I describe a few elements of Brain Gym that you can introduce quickly and easily in the classroom.

Just Add Water

The first technique for maximizing brain function is simply to drink plenty of ordinary water, at least a quart a day per hundred pounds of body weight. In times of stress it may be wise to double or triple that amount. Aside from its other health benefits, water maintains the electrolytic balance in the nerve cells, without which they can't transmit impulses effectively. Coffee, tea, alcohol, some carbonated drinks, and chocolate, on the other hand, tend to lead to an electrolyte imbalance. Carla Hannaford's book *Smart Moves* (1995, 138) gives a good deal of technical detail I won't reiterate here, but keep in mind the value of that humble glass of water.

Cross Crawl

This activity doesn't involve crawling at all. Rather, it involves walking in place, lifting each knee high enough to touch the opposite elbow to it, right elbow to left knee and vice versa (see figure 5-2). This exercise helps to enhance nerve activity

Study Skills, Self-Management, and Conflict Resolution

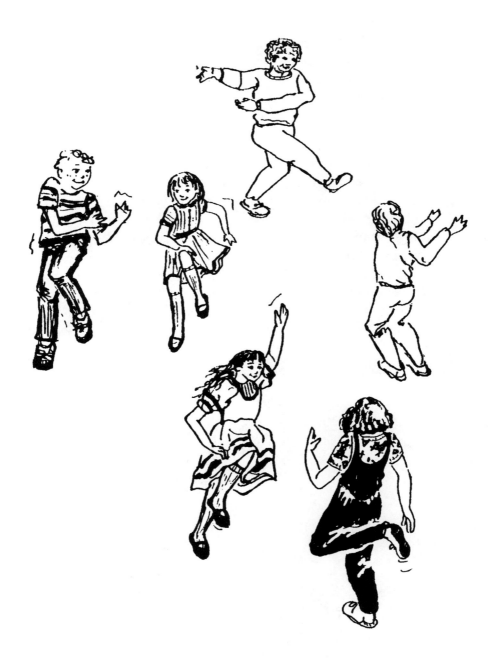

Figure 5-2. Cross crawl

Chapter 5

across the corpus callosum. Done regularly, the activity helps form more nerve networks, allowing better communication between the hemispheres for higher-order thinking. You might want to play some music and have students make up their own dances based on this pattern.

Lazy Eights

You can do this activity as a writing or eye exercise. As a writing exercise, this large-muscle activity helps promote the rhythm and flow that improve hand-eye coordination. Done with a pencil and paper, it can help relieve writer's block or simply improve handwriting. Since it is done with both hands and involves crossing the midline of the body, it also helps promote neural development across the hemispheres. Use a chalkboard or a large piece of paper on a table or taped to a wall. Draw a sideways figure eight (infinity symbol), beginning at the center and moving up to the left

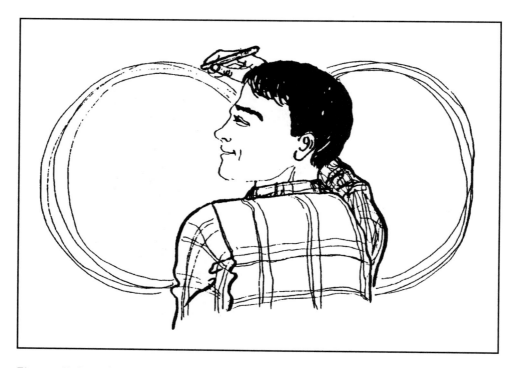

Figure 5-3. Lazy eights

(counterclockwise), then over and around (see figure 5-3). Make five or more lazy eights with each hand, then five with both hands together, each one holding a pencil.

Done as an eye exercise, lazy eights can strengthen the extrinsic eye muscles and improve neural network development for fine motor tracking to improve reading. For those who use computers often, it can help relieve the stress of gazing at the monitor for long periods. Hold your thumb at eye level about an elbow's distance from your nose. Slowly and smoothly, move the thumb through the lazy eight pattern, keeping the head relaxed but still and following the thumb with the eyes. Repeat at least three times with each hand. Then repeat using both hands clasped together with the thumbs forming an *x*.

The Elephant

This exercise helps enhance overall balance and integration. In a standing position with knees relaxed, tilt your head so your left ear touches your left shoulder. Keeping it in that position, stretch your left arm in front of you like an elephant's trunk. Trace a lazy eight pattern in the air several times; then repeat, tilting your head right and using the right arm. This exercise helps activate the vestibular system for balance, the basal ganglia, cerebellum, and the sensory and motor areas of the cerebrum. It has been found very helpful with people who experience attention difficulties (see figure 5-4).

Self-Management

As I mentioned in chapter 1, internal sensing and self-calming are a key to self-regulating behavior. Detailed instructions for introducing these skills appear in chapter 1. In this chapter, I build on the basics and show how you can refine these psychophysical techniques and apply them to conflict resolution.

The techniques in this section are adapted from ones in *Mastery* and other books by George Leonard.

Chapter 5

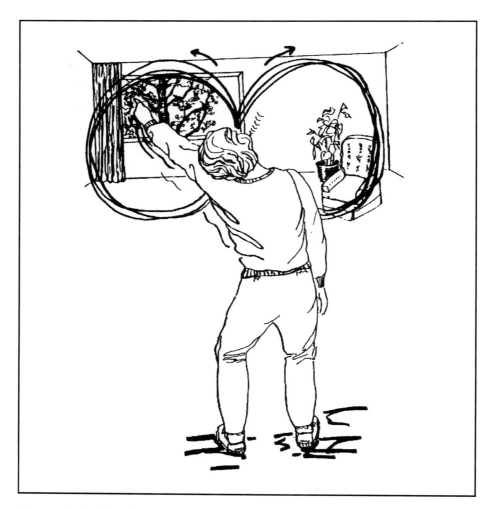

Figure 5-4. The elephant

Returning to Center

This activity (from page 158 of *Mastery*) demonstrates to students that they can return to a centered state and even deepen it after an interruption.

Optional Script

You probably remember that we've practiced a way that you can calm yourself when you feel stressed. Sometimes it's referred to as being centered. Many martial artists practice being centered as much as they practice the other techniques of their art. A story is told about one of the greatest martial artists of this century, Morihei Ueshiba, the founder of aikido. Even as a man in his seventies, he could throw four or five burly attackers at once. People often asked him how he could always be centered in the midst of rapid multiple attacks. He replied, "I'm not always centered. I get off center very often. I simply return to center before anyone notices." This story is part of the oral tradition in aikido dojos.

We're going to practice getting centered, then doing things to interrupt that calm alertness, which will give us a chance to practice returning to center. Sometimes it's possible to get to a state of even deeper calmness and alertness after an interruption.

Stand next to your desks with your feet about shoulder width apart. Let your feet feel well balanced on the floor. Breathe deeply and comfortably, as if the breath can go all the way to your center. Let your belly and your back relax without slumping. Your arms are hanging comfortably at your sides. As you breathe, you feel your body and mind are balanced, relaxed, and alert at the same time. Let yourself be grounded, relaxed, aware, centered, and energized.

Now, close your eyes and gently let yourself slump forward from the waist. Your knees can bend a bit, and your arms and your head can hang down limply, like those of a rag doll. When I clap my hands, straighten yourself up rather quickly and open your eyes. Clap and give students time to straighten up.

You're probably feeling a little disoriented. Don't fight against that feeling. Experience it completely, but touch your center with one hand and let yourself settle into a balanced and centered state again. Remember the shortcut word: grace. You're grounded, relaxed, aware, centered, and energized. Be aware of all that happened in this process. See if you feel more deeply centered than you did before the interruption.

A variation of this exercise is to have students open their eyes and spin around several times—just enough to get a little dizzy. Then they return to center, placing special attention on a sense of groundedness in the soles of their feet.

Drawing Energy from Unexpected Blows

This activity from Leonard (1992, 160) requires a reasonable amount of open space in order to allow students to practice with a partner.

Optional Script

Sometimes life gives us nasty surprises. Maybe it's a D on a quiz, a broken date, or even worse, a serious injury or the loss of someone we love. Struggling blindly against a misfortune can pull you further away from center. On the other hand, acting as though you were made of steel and denying the pain and shock can make you brittle or numb. Even worse, feeling sorry for yourself and doing nothing but whining can turn you into a self-pitying wimp.

There's something else you can do, though. With practice, you can gain energy from a serious misfortune. In a way, it's like taking the hit as a gift. We'll practice it with a physical activity, then you might consider how you can apply the idea to other situations.

I'll demonstrate first, then you'll have a chance to practice with a partner. May I have a volunteer to be my partner? Choose a reliable volunteer. *I'm going to stand here, and I'd like my partner to stand slightly behind me. Keeping my eyes open, I'll quietly center myself. When I'm feeling centered, I'll hold my arms out at about a forty-five degree angle.* (See figure 5-5.) *That will be a signal for my partner to come up and grab one of my wrists rather tightly with two hands and hold on—not tightly enough to hurt, but enough to represent a sudden blow.* (See figure 5-6.)

Instead of struggling against the blow or pretending it's not a shock, I'll try to be fully aware of how it affected me. I'll describe it aloud, with plenty of detail. For example, I might say, "I jumped slightly and felt a shot of adrenaline. My heart is beating faster. I feel the muscles in that arm tensing." If I feel tight in any part of me, I'll just tighten it a little more to become fully aware of it. My partner will keep holding on while I continue describing how I feel to give me practice in facing a real blow squarely and being aware of how I really feel about it.

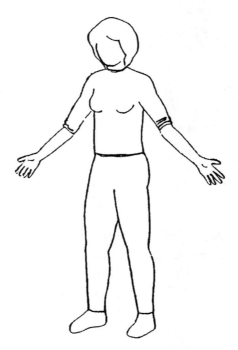

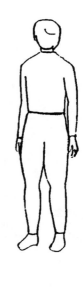

Figure 5-5. Preparing to draw energy from unexpected blows

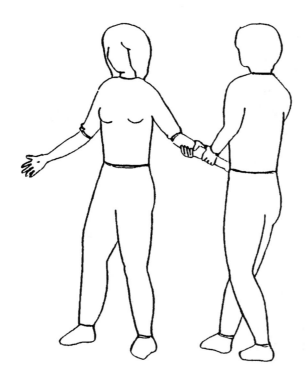

Figure 5-6. Drawing energy from unexpected blows

> *Then I'll bend my knees just a little to help me get back into a balanced and centered state. My partner will keep holding my wrist. I will feel that the grab actually gives me energy that can help me deal with the situation. It won't solve the problem by itself, but it can give me the physical energy, the awareness, and the will to deal with the problem. I'll take some deep, relaxed breaths and feel the clarity filling my body. I'll shake my hands slightly, the signal for my partner to let go. I'll feel the energy expanding, then walk around a bit, as if I'm expanding too, as if I can use the energy to deal with the problem.*

Demonstrate to students, then have them find partners and try it themselves. In a follow-up discussion, find out how people reacted. Once students have learned the basic technique, they can practice applying it to a problem. Have them begin by thinking of a problem, real or imaginary. Ask them to describe it in a few sentences or in a quick drawing. Ask them to imagine that the grab represents the problem they've chosen. After completing the exercise, ask them to write or draw the steps toward solution that presented themselves.

Relaxing for Power

You can demonstrate or have students fully participate in this activity, which is adapted from Leonard (1992, 164). If you'd like students to participate, be sure you have enough space for them.

Optional Script

Let's experiment with power—your own power, not the stuff that comes from engines or electric outlets. The word power *comes from French and Latin roots that mean "to be able." In its original meaning, power is not domination over others, but your own ability to do things. You may already know that a rigid muscle tends to lose strength and that real muscular power is related to an alert state of relaxation. After we demonstrate this phenomenon physically, I'd like you to think of how it might work in your approach to life in general.*

I'd like a volunteer to help me demonstrate. Choose a reliable volunteer. I'm going to stand and hold my right arm out in front. We could use either arm, but this time we'll use the right. I have my hand open with my thumb up and fingers spread. My partner will stand to the right of my arm and bend it at the elbow by pressing up on my wrist and down on my elbow. I'm not going to resist this time; I'll just let my arm bend. (See figure 5-7.)

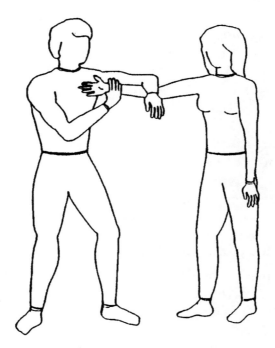

Figure 5-7. Relaxing for power

Now I'm going to try two different ways of making my arm strong so it will be harder to bend. My partner will try to bend it just as before, adding force gradually. This isn't a contest. It's just a way of comparing two ways of being powerful.

My first way is to hold my arm very rigid. I'll tighten all my muscles and try to make it very hard for my partner to bend my arm. It may or may not actually bend, but I need to notice how much effort I exert to keep my arm as straight as possible. I also need to notice how it feels to me when I do it. Now partner, try to bend my arm, and pay attention to how much effort you have to put into it, and how you feel as you do it . . .

Next, I'll try it in a different way. I'll center myself and hold my arm out in the same way. This time I feel energy flowing from my shoulder to my fingertips, and I imagine my arm as part of a thick, immensely powerful laser beam that goes out through my fingertips, through the walls, and all the way to the end of the universe. My arm isn't rigid, but it isn't limp, either. It's full of life and energy, surrounded by that laser beam. When my partner tries to bend my arm, the energy will become even more powerful.

Now, partner, apply the same amount of pressure that you did before, and notice how you feel this time . . .

After trying the second time, share your observations. The majority of people who try this experiment find that the second way is much more powerful than the first. Electromyographic measurements have actually shown that the second way produces more strength in the arm. Moreover, people usually find that the second way feels more harmonious than the first. If time and space allow, have students work as partners and try the experiment for themselves. Follow with a discussion. Remind them that they can try the same approach in other aspects of their lives, using a relaxed, alert, assertive attitude rather than a rigid, combative one. It's possible to be strong, relaxed, and gentle at the same time.

Conflict Resolution: A Mind and Body Matter

The secret of successful conflict resolution is to be strong and gentle, self-respecting and respectful of others, at the same time. Several kinesthetic activities help achieve this state of being. As I discuss preparation and techniques for conflict resolution, I mention physical activities that help. I have introduced some already; I describe others in detail at the end of the chapter.

What Is Conflict?

Conflict is an interference pattern of energies. It's a fact of life, neither good nor bad, just inevitable. In fact, growth is not a possibility unless some form of conflict exists. Many conflict resolution ideas in this section come from Terry Dobson's *Giving in to Get Your Way*. He points out that we can't eliminate conflict, but we can change our response to it so that it's more likely to turn out positively.

Conflict generally has three possible outcomes:

1. Win/Lose: This outcome is what we generally expect when we think of conflict. One side wins and one loses. Most athletic contests are structured this way, but life isn't necessarily so.

2. Lose/Lose: Many conflicts result in everyone's losing in one way or another, especially when the conflict is handled clumsily. A bitter fight over child custody is an example.

3. Win/Win: In this third situation, a conflict that is handled skillfully results in everyone's winning in some way. The pioneering work done by people such as Terry Dobson has led to increased use of a win/win approach. Labor-management negotiations are often structured to aim at a win/win outcome.

Getting Ready to Resolve Conflict

A key to gaining a win/win resolution is proper preparation. Following are several steps.

1. Recognize that a conflict exists and articulate it clearly. Conflict won't usually go away if you pretend it doesn't exist. On the other hand, if you acknowledge it clearly, you can decide how to deal with it, which might include ignoring it. The activity called "Drawing Energy from Unexpected Blows," found earlier in this chapter, is a good physical metaphor for acknowledging and describing a conflict.

2. Evaluate the possible outcomes. Must the outcome be win/lose? Might it be lose/lose? Could it be win/win?

3. Evaluate the parties involved. Take into account both the verbal and nonverbal messages on all sides. Evaluate your own position and that of the people with whom you are in conflict.

Yourself

Either as a participant or as a mediator, knowing your own state of mind and body is crucial.

- Are you centered? Do a quick check. You may need to go through the process of "Internal Sensing and Self-Calming." You might even want to practice the exercise called "Relaxing for Power." If you feel too much anger, try one of the techniques listed in the "Choosing Techniques for Resolution" section.

- Be sure you feel respect for yourself *and* for the others involved. A good physical activity to demonstrate whether you feel respectful is the "Wimpo, Macho, and Mensch Solve a Problem" activity from earlier in this chapter.

- Check on whether you feel a sense of concern and are flexible about the outcome. Being willing to accept only one specific solution can undermine genuine resolution efforts.

The Person with Whom You Are In Conflict

- Determine who the person really is. Keep in mind that human beings of all ages may be skillful at manipulating and making someone else look guilty.

- What is the person's state of mind? Is she too angry to talk? If that's the case, you may need to postpone the resolution or use a technique that doesn't require rational talking.

- What is your relationship with that person? Is the conflict with a stranger on a bus whom you'll never see again, or is it with a family member, colleague, or close friend? Keep in mind that relationships are always changing anyway and that you can take charge of the direction of change.

4. Evaluate the time and place. Do you need privacy? Keep in mind that no communication happens when any participants are playing for an audience. Consider whether you have enough time to resolve the issue and whether anyone involved needs cooling-off time.

Choosing Techniques for Resolution

You may decide to use one or more of these suggestions.

- Discuss the issue politely and firmly. Be sure you're using "I" messages. Rather than saying "You made me angry," try saying "I felt angry when you did that." In the classroom, you may want to have students practice saying "I" messages to one another, and also focus on the next suggestion.

  Avoid using absolutes such as *always* and *never*. You may be amazed at how difficult it is because our everyday conversation includes absolutes so often. There's a solid, practical reason for avoiding them, however. It's almost impossible to be accurate if you use absolutes. Virtually no one *always* does something or *never* does something. Using absolutes leaves you open to being refuted logically. Instead, you might try such phrases as "often" or "hardly ever."

  Be sure you have a balance of attention: you're genuinely hearing the other person's point of view. (You might try the physical activity called "Silent Talking and Listening" at the end of this chapter.) At the same time, you're fully aware of any hogwash and not letting it knock you off center. (Students can practice this awareness with "The Gift Game," also at the end of this chapter.) Refer to rules already established and understood if they're applicable.

- Defuse excess anger. If anyone involved is too angry to talk, you might suggest a cooling-off time. Other ways include the following:

    breathing deeply and comfortably

    hitting a pillow

    exercising vigorously

    talking quietly with a respected friend

- Request a mediator. Remind students that asking for a mediator isn't the same as tattling. It's simply a civilized way to find a solution that works for everyone. The mediator may be a teacher, a peer, or another reliable person. Following are some guidelines for a smooth mediation process:

    Mediator takes notes, if possible.

    Participants talk to one another, not mediator.

    Participants follow the guidelines for the technique "Discuss the issue politely and firmly."

    Participants take turns talking with no interruptions.

    Participants repeat turns, if necessary.

    Mediator asks for observations from others who have witnessed the situation.

    Participants share afterward how they could have handled the situation differently.

    Participants offer solutions and appropriate consequences. Be prepared to suggest some if the participants don't suggest any.

    Decide on a follow-up process to see that the issue is resolved.

- It may be appropriate to do nothing. Sometimes the conflict is too absurd to merit attention, or the person with whom you're in conflict isn't worth worrying about. After evaluating it, you may decide that it's best to do nothing at all. Sometimes letting go is hard to do because you fear you may appear cowardly. The activity called "Refusing a Challenge" at the end of this chapter is a good practice.

At other times, you may choose to do nothing in the present, which allows you to change the time and place of resolution, or to surprise the other person and invite a new perspective.

- Withdraw physically. Of course, if you're facing physical danger, your best approach is probably to escape, if possible. Sometimes there are other reasons for choosing this option. For instance, you can withdraw temporarily to allow for a better time and place to resolve the issue. Sometimes you can withdraw permanently if there are no other options. Keep in mind that this withdrawal will probably result in a drastic change in lifestyle. When discussing this option with students, it's wise to point out that it has to be used very sparingly. A lot of misery comes from the extreme forms of withdrawal: running away from home, drug involvement, divorce, child abandonment, and suicide. Most problems are *not* solved by attempts to permanently withdrawal.

- Do the unexpected to give a new perspective. Introducing humor, imagination, or genuine vulnerability sometimes opens possibilities for resolution. A farcical but applicable literary example is Petruchio in *The Taming of the Shrew*. The story of Brer Rabbit and the briar patch is another analogy.

- Restore harmony with positive feelings. This option requires a good deal of skill. It's the topic of many stories of great religious leaders. Historically, it was used effectively by people such as Gandhi and Martin Luther King Jr. A recent example can be found in a true story, "A Kind Answer" by Terry Dobson (1985).

Role-Playing Everyday Conflicts and Resolutions

After students have been introduced to the elements of conflict resolution, you can ask them to suggest types of everyday conflicts and make up skits to show several alternative solutions: win/lose, lose/lose, and win/win. They may use one conflict resolution technique or several.

More Physical Activities for Conflict Resolution

Silent Talking and Listening

This activity is adapted from Leonard's *Leonard Energy Training* (1983, 155). To demonstrate this activity, you need enough space so you and a partner can walk back and forth about fifteen or twenty feet. To have an entire class practice the activity in partners, you need an appropriate amount of open space.

Optional Script

Communication isn't just a matter of words; it involves your entire being. In a way, each time we communicate, we express what we are. There's a saying, "What you are speaks so loudly that I cannot hear your words." That's what we'll be exploring in this activity. Instead of using words, you'll communicate with your being. Your communication will be expressed in a simple physical activity. I'll need a volunteer to help me demonstrate. Choose a reliable volunteer.

I'll stand directly in front of my partner, about two feet away. Now I'm going to move to my left a little, so my right foot is just to the right of my partner's right foot. I'll place my hand on my partner's upper chest so that my thumb and index finger form a "V" just where the neck and upper chest meet. You notice that I'm not putting my hand on my partner's neck. That could get dangerous. (See figure 5-8.)

For this activity, walking forward symbolizes talking, and walking backward signifies listening. Each of us will take turns doing both. Just for this experiment, whether we're walking forward or backward, my partner and I are not going to look at each other. Of course, when you're really talking to someone, it's

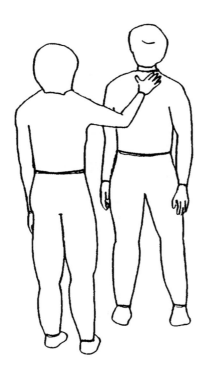

Figure 5-8. Silent talking and listening

often best to make eye contact, but for this activity, we'll communicate just with body movement.

When I say, "Begin," we'll start walking. I'll keep my hand on my partner's upper chest and walk forward. My partner will walk backward. For this first try, I'd like my partner to convey an attitude of resisting what I have to say. Partner, please do this by leaning into my hand, using just enough resistance to make me struggle to move you back. You'll point your resistance straight forward instead of moving sideways so that neither of us will lose our balance. I'll walk forward in a straight line and stop before we run into anything. Okay, begin. Move forward silently about fifteen or twenty feet, as your partner moves backward, resisting your pressure. Pause a few seconds.

I'm thinking about how it felt to try to communicate with someone who seemed to resist everything I was "saying." I'd like my partner to reflect on how it felt to resist everything I said.

Now we'll reverse roles. Partner, you'll put your hand on my upper chest and become the "talker," and I'll be the resistant "listener." When I say, "Begin," you'll move forward and I'll resist you as I move backward to the place where we started. Okay, begin. Walk as partners, you backward and your partner forward, back to the place where you began. Pause a few seconds for reflection. Then repeat the process a time or two.

Now we'll try the same kind of communication in a different mode. This time, the listening partner will convey an attitude of not paying attention or not caring. Of course, the partner knows someone is trying to communicate, but isn't interested in what's being said. It's as if I were talking to someone who keeps saying "uh-huh," without really hearing what I'm saying. Have any of you ever known someone who does that? To tell the truth, we probably all do that now and then.

Partner, you'll symbolize this inattentive way of being by leaning back just a little during the walking, so that there's not really any contact between my hand and your chest. When I say "Begin," we'll start walking and you'll stay just slightly ahead of my hand, but neither of us will go too fast. We don't want to make this into a chase game. Okay, begin. Walk forward as your partner walks backward just a little ahead of your contact. Stop after fifteen or twenty feet, pause a second or two, and reverse roles. After one or two times of going back and forth in this mode, pause for a few seconds for reflection.

Now, we'll try a third way. This time, partner, you're going to convey an attitude of real interest in what I have to say. You won't arbitrarily resist or let your attention drift. Take a moment to balance and center yourself and I'll do the same. When I walk forward, you'll move backward in a way that keeps up a gentle and firm contact with my hand. Your movement will tell me that you're totally present, caring about me and what I say. Okay, begin. Walk forward as before, pause a second or two, then reverse roles as before. Repeat the process a few times, then stop. Ask your partner for his or her reflections on each mode of communication. Invite the others to give their observations. Then have students pair up to try it themselves. Have the pairs of partners walk in parallel lines so they don't bump into one another. Repeat the instructions as students go through each mode of communication.

How did it feel in that last mode of communication? Was it different from the first two? . . . Think about whether you usually communicate in one of these three ways when you're talking to your friends . . . Is it different when you're talking to people in your family? . . . How about when you're on a date? . . . Which way of communication would you want to use in a job interview? . . . Remember that you have a choice.

The Gift Game

This activity, adapted from Patterson and Wortz (1977, 26) gives students a different perspective on teasing or insults.

Optional Script

Sometimes someone says something that you know is false or exaggerated. Sometimes a person may try to put you down or call you a name. You don't have to accept their words. You don't even have to get upset. This activity is one way of practicing being centered when someone says something upsetting.

Hold out your hands as if you had a gift-wrapped box in them. Then turn toward one of the students. *I have something for you. It's a box of South American poison-dart toads that can kill you with just one tiny touch. Would you like to open it?* The student may or may not say anything, but will probably indicate some reluctance.

Feel free to say, "No, thank you." You don't have to accept it, and you don't have to get upset. The box belongs to the person who is offering it. Just tell me politely that you don't want it, and it stays with me. Go to several of the students, offering the gift box with a different negative gift each time. Use your imagination or consult the list following this script for items to put in the box. Encourage each person to refuse politely.

The things people say to you are like gifts, but they're not always the kind you want to accept. Now I'm going to give each of you a chance to offer someone else a gift. Have students practice offering and refusing gifts with partners.

When you're trying to work out a conflict with someone, that person may say something that's not true or something that's exaggerated or downright rotten. Just silently say, "No, thank you." You can even quietly shake your head, but keep breathing comfortably. If you feel yourself tightening up, let those muscles tighten a tiny bit more, then relax them. Then when it's your turn to talk, you'll still be centered and you can present your side of the issue effectively.

Suggestions for the "Gift Box"

rock-bottom SAT scores

runny noses

malarial mosquitoes

D's and F's

athlete's foot

a case of food poisoning

Saturday nights without dates

black widow spiders

Refusing a Challenge

This activity, used by George Leonard in his seminars, helps students to practice ignoring minor conflicts such as teasing or name-calling. Please emphasize, though, that it may not work for handling a physical threat.

One student walks up to another and issues a silent challenge by raising his right fist to represent teasing or name-calling. The student who has been challenged stands solidly, meeting the gaze of the challenger with a calm facial expression. After breathing comfortably a few times, the challenged student turns away from the challenger and, keeping that sense of solidity, walks off as if nothing had happened. Ask each participant to tell how the experience felt. The rest of the students take turns as partners, then discuss their reactions.

Appendix

KEY	
Eng =	English and Second Language
M&S =	Math and Science
SS =	Social Studies
St&S =	Study Skills and Self-Management
Kin imag =	Kinesthetic Imagination

Cross-Referenced Chart of Activities

Activity	Category	Eng	M&S	SS	St&S	Page
Acting Out Word Problems	Whole Body		X			72
Algebra Project	All		X			70
Amendment Boogie	Whole Body			X		54
"Baking" Cookies	Hands-on	X				36
Blind Date	Whole Body	X				38
Centering	Large Muscle				X	16
Cerebellar Minestrone	Whole Body				X	92
Civil War Simulation	Whole Body			X		60
Computer Math Games	Hands-on		X			72
Conflict Resolution	Whole Body	X		X	X	112
Cooperative Group Work	All	X	X	X	X	14
Cross Crawl	Whole Body	X	X	X	X	102
Cross-Sensing	Kin Imag	X			X	100
Designing a House	Hands-on	X	X	X		74
Economics Simulations	Hands-on			X		63
Elephant	Large Muscle	X	X	X	X	105
Energy from Unexpected Blows	Whole Body	X	X	X	X	108
Escape from Srebrenica	Kin Imag	X		X		64
Geography Simulations	Hands-on			X		63
Getting into the Historical Picture	Whole Body			X		45
Getting into the Literary Picture	Whole Body	X				27
Gift Game	Hands-on	X		X	X	121

Cross-Referenced Chart of Activities

Activity	Category	Eng	M&S	SS	St&S	Page
Historical Museum	Hands-on			X		56
History Celebrity Party	Whole Body			X		45
Human Continuum	Whole Body	X	X	X		44
Human Graph	Whole Body	X	X	X		43
Imaginary Journey: History	Kin Imag			X		44
Imaginary Journey: Literature	Kin Imag	X				25
Imaginary Journey: Science	Kin Imag		X			75
Impersonations: History	Whole Body			X		45
Impersonations: Literary	Whole Body	X				26
Informal Dramatics: History	Whole Body			X		45
Informal Dramatics: Literature	Whole Body	X				26
Interactive Slide Lecture	Whole Body	X		X		55
Internal Sensing/Self-Calming	Large Muscle	X	X	X	X	16
Interplanetary Distances	Whole Body		X			78
Inventing U.S. Government	Hands-on			X		46
Journey Inside an Atom	Kin Imag		X			87
Kent State Simulation	Whole Body			X		57
Kinesthetic Imagination	Kin Imag	X	X	X	X	19
Kinesthetic Shakespeare	Whole Body	X				28
Lazy Eights	Large Muscle	X			X	104
Literary Celebrity Party	Whole Body	X				26
Magic Lamp	Hands-on	X				38
Manipulative Math materials	Hands-on		X			73
Map Puzzles of Continents	Hands-on			X		61
Math Celebrity Party	Whole Body		X			74
Math Simulation Game	Hands-on		X			74
McCarthyism in 1950s	Whole Body			X		55
Models and Dioramas	Hands-on	X	X	X		30
Paragraph or Essay Ad Libs	Whole Body	X				34
People Maps	Whole Body			X		62
Personal Expert Trainer	Whole Body	X	X	X	X	94

Cross-Referenced Chart of Activities

Activity	Category	Eng	M&S	SS	St&S	Page
Picture Derby	Hands-on	X	X	X		31
Punctuation Sounds and Actions	Large Muscle	X				33
Raps	Large Muscle	X	X	X		27
Refusing a Challenge	Whole Body	X		X	X	122
Relaxing for Power	Large Muscle				X	110
Restaurant	Whole Body	X				37
Returning to Center	Whole Body				X	106
Science Museum	Hands-on		X			76
Science Simulations	Hands-on		X			77
Scientific Celebrity Party	Whole Body		X			75
Scientific Skits	Whole Body		X			76
Self-Calming (Centering)	Large Muscle	X	X	X	X	16
Sentence Ad Libs	Whole Body	X				34
Service Learning	Whole Body	X	X	X	X	22
Shooting Math Baskets	Large Muscle		X			74
Sign Language Alphabet	Hands-on	X	X	X		30
Silent Talking & Listening	Whole Body	X		X	X	118
Solar Wind, Plasma	Whole Body		X			79
Soup Kitchen Simulation	Whole Body	X		X		57
Superwhammo	Whole Body	X				39
Tech Terms Rondo Rap	Small Muscle	X	X	X		76
Total Physical Response	Whole Body	X				34
Trenches of WWI simulation	Whole Body	X		X		55
Trial in History	Whole Body			X		60
Trip to Shakespeare's England	Kin Imag	X		X		40
Verb Form Charades	Whole Body	X				31
Vocabulary Charades	Whole Body	X				31
Whole-Body Geometry	Whole Body		X			72
Wimpo, Macho, & Mench	Whole Body	X			X	98
Working on Assembly Line simulation	Hands-on			X		55
Write on What??	Hands-on	X				31

Bibliography

Multiple Intelligences

Armstrong, T. 1993. *Seven Kinds of Smart: Identifying and Developing Your Many Intelligences.* New York: Penguin.

———. 1994. *Multiple Intelligences in the Classroom.* Alexandria, Va.: Association for Supervision and Curriculum Development.

Bruetsch, A. 1994. *Multiple Intelligences Lesson Plan Book.* Tucson, Ariz.: Zephyr Press.

Campbell, L., B. Campbell, and D. Dickinson. 1992. *Teaching and Learning through Multiple Intelligences.* Seattle, Wash.: New Horizons for Learning.

Chapman, C. 1993. *If the Shoe Fits . . . How to Develop Multiple Intelligences in the Classroom.* Palatine, Ill.: Skylight.

Gardner, Howard. 1983. *Frames of Mind: The Theory of Multiple Intelligences.* New York: Basic.

———. 1993. *Multiple Intelligences: The Theory in Practice.* New York, Basic.

Ghiselin, B. 1952. *The Creative Process.* Berkeley: U. of California Press.

Lazear, D. 1991a. *Seven Ways of Knowing.* Palatine, Ill.: Skylight.

———. 1991b. *Seven Ways of Teaching.* Palatine, Ill.: Skylight.

———. 1994a. *Multiple Intelligence Approaches to Assessment.* Tucson, Ariz.: Zephyr Press.

———. 1994b. *Seven Pathways of Learning: Teaching Students and Parents about Multiple Intelligences.* Tucson, Ariz.: Zephyr Press.

Bibliography

Margulies, N. 1995. *The Magic Seven: Tools for Building Your Multiple Intelligences.* Tucson, Ariz.: Zephyr Press.

New City School. 1994. *Celebrating Multiple Intelligences.* St. Louis: New City School Press.

Bodily-Kinesthetic Intelligence

Benzwie, T. 1988. *A Moving Experience: Dance for Lovers of Children and the Child Within.* Tucson, Ariz.: Zephyr Press.

———. 1996. *More Moving Experiences: Connecting the Arts, Feelings, and Imagination.* Tucson, Ariz.: Zephyr Press.

Grant, J. 1995. *Shake, Rattle, and Learn: Classroom-Tested Ideas That Use Movement for Active Learning.* York, Maine: Stenhouse.

Griss, S. 1994. "Creative Movement: A Language for Learning" *Educational Leadership* 51, no. 5 (February): 78.

Hannaford, C. 1993. *Education in Motion: A Practical Guide to Whole-Brain Body Integration for Everyone.* Video. Available from Zephyr Press.

———. 1995. *Smart Moves: Why Learning Is Not All in Your Head.* Arlington, Va.: Great Ocean Publishers.

Herman, G., and P. Hollingsworth. 1992. *Kinetic Kaleidoscope: Exploring Movement and Energy in the Visual Arts.* Tucson, Ariz.: Zephyr Press.

English and Second Languages

Asher, J. 1993. *Learning Another Language through Actions.* Los Gatos, Calif.: Sky Oaks Productions, Inc. Available from Berty Segal, Inc. 1749 Eucalyptus St., Brea, CA 92621, (714) 529-5359.

Flachmann, M. Forthcoming. "Suit the Action to the Word: Teaching Minds and Bodies in the College Classroom" in *Inspired Teaching,* ed. by John Roth. Bolton, Mass.: Anker Press.

Galyean, B. 1984. *Language from Within.* Tucson, Ariz.: Center for Integrative Learning.

Krashen, S., and T. Terrell. 1983. *The Natural Approach: Language Acquisition in the Classroom.* Englewood Cliffs, N.J.: Prentice-Hall. Available from Berty Segal Inc. 1749 Eucalyptus St., Brea, CA 92621, (714) 529-5359.

National Association for the Deaf. American Sign Language Manual Alphabet. (Poster.) 814 Thayer Avenue, Silver Spring, MD 20910.

Patterson, M. 1989. *Shakespeare for Kids*. Bakersfield, Calif.: Patterson Learning Services. Series of ten Shakespeare plays adapted for elementary and middle school students, accompanied by activities for multiple intelligences. Available from publisher. P. O. Box 2206, Bakersfield, CA 93303, (805) 833-0453.

Segal, B. 1995. *Teaching English through Action*. Brea, Calif.: Berty Segal Inc. Total Physical Response method. Available from the publisher. 1749 Eucalyptus St., Brea, CA 92621, (714) 529-5359.

Shope, R. 1995. *Mime Writing*. Whittier: Calif.: Mime Media Instructional Technologies. Using interactive video and simple mime techniques to teach language arts. Available through the publisher. P. O. Box 4225, Whittier, CA 90607, (310) 693-9053.

Social Sciences

Fritz, Jean. 1987. *Shh! We're Writing the Constitution*. New York: Scholastic Inc.

Interact. A wide range of classroom simulation games, such as "Depression Soup Kitchen," "Kent State Tragedy," "Trials in History," "Civil War," "Sanga," "Boxcars," and "Pacific Rim," for middle school and high school social sciences. 1825 Gillespie Way 101-A, El Cajon, CA 92020, (800) 359-0961.

Jones, Richard. 1996. *Gumshoe Geography: Exploring the Cultural, Physical, Sociological, and Biological Characteristics of Our Planet*. Tucson, Ariz.: Zephyr Press.

Selwyn, D. 1993. *Living History in the Classroom*. Tucson Ariz.: Zephyr Press.

Smithsonian Institution. 1993. *Resource Guide for Teachers*. Washington, D.C.: Smithsonian Institution. Up to nine copies available for free from the publisher. Office of Secondary and Elementary Education, Smithsonian Institution, Arts and Industries Building, Room 1163, MRC 402, Washington, D.C. 20560, (202) 357-2425.

Bibliography

Teachers' Curriculum Institute. 1994. *History Alive! Engaging All Learners in the Diverse Classroom*. Menlo Park, Calif.: Addison-Wesley. Available from Teachers' Curriculum Institute. 4149 El Camino Way, Ste B, Palo Alto, CA 94306-4010, (800) 497-6138.

———. 1996. *History Alive! Professional Development Video Program*. New York: Addison-Wesley. Available from Zephyr Press.

Mathematics and Natural Sciences

Barkman, R. 1994. *Coaching Science Stars*. Tucson, Ariz.: Zephyr Press.

Bulla, Dale. 1996. *Think Math! Interactive Loops for Groups*. Tucson, Ariz.: Zephyr Press.

Davidson & Associates. *Math Blaster: Mystery* and *Alge-Blaster*. Computer programs for pre-algebra and algebra, for Windows or Macintosh. Available from Davidson & Associates, Inc. P. O. Box 2961, Torrance, CA 90509, (800) 545-7677.

Erickson, T. 1989. *Get It Together: Math Problems for Groups, Grades 4-12*. Berkeley: University of California, Lawrence Hall of Science. Available from Zephyr Press.

Glencoe/McGraw-Hill. 1995. *Interactive Mathematics: Activities and Investigations*. New York: Glencoe/McGraw-Hill.

Hiner, M. 1985. *Paper Engineering for Pop-up Books and Cards*. Norfolk, England: Tarquin Productions. Available from Zephyr Press.

Interact. Classroom simulation games such as *Math Quest, Checkbook, Galaxy, Future Quest, Balance,* and *Clone*. Available from Interact, 1825 Gillespie Way 101-A, El Cajon, CA 92020, (800) 359-0961.

Jagoda, J. et al. N.d. *Shapes, Loops, and Images: Exhibit Guide*. Berkeley, Calif.: Lawrence Hall of Science.

Laurence Hall of Science. N.d. *To Build a House: GEMS and the Thematic Approach to Teaching Science*. Berkeley: University of California. Available from the publisher. Berkeley, CA 94720, (510) 642-7771.

Montessori Manipulative Materials. Available from Village Faire for Educators. 10594 Combie Rd. 106515, Auburn, CA 95603, (916) 268-0607.

Pethoud, R. 1993. *Pi in the Sky: Hands-on Mathematical Activities for Teaching Astronomy.* Tucson, Ariz: Zephyr Press.

Pluto Express Educational Outreach Materials. NASA/Jet Propulsion Laboratory, Richard Shope, Curriculum Development Lead. Curriculum guides and videotape available to schools at no cost from NASA/JPL, Pluto Express Educational Outreach, Mail Stop 301-250D, 4800 Oak Grove Drive, Pasadena, CA 91109, (818) 354-3812. E-mail address: pluto.education@jpl.nasa.gov.

Shope, R. 1993. *Teaching Math Mimediately.* Whittier, Calif.: Mime Media Instructional Technologies. Available from the publisher. P. O. Box 4225, Whittier, CA 90607, (310) 693-9053.

Smithsonian Institution. 1993. *Resource Guide for Teachers.* Washington, D.C.: Smithsonian Institution. Lists about 400 free and inexpensive items available from several museums and organizations: posters, slides, video and audio tapes, etc. Up to nine copies free from the publisher. Office of Secondary and Elementary Education, Smithsonian Institution, Arts and Industries Building, Room 1163, MRC 402, Washington, D.C. 20560, (202) 357-2425.

Stenmark, J., Thompson, V., and Cossey, R. 1986. *Family Math.* Berkeley: University of California, Lawrence Hall of Science. Available from Zephyr Press.

Thompson, F. 1994. *Hands-on Math! Ready-to-Use Games and Activities for Grades 4-8.* West Nyack, New York: Center for Applied Research in Education. Available from Zephyr Press.

Uribe, D. 1993. *Fractal Cuts: Exploring the Magic of Fractals with Pop-up Designs.* Norfolk, England: Tarquin Productions.

Watson, Bruce. 1992. "If a = Math and b = Magic, Then $a + b$ = The Algebra Project." *Smithsonian* (February): 114.

Bibliography

Study Skills, Self-Management, and Conflict Resolution

Crum, T. 1987. *The Magic of Conflict.* New York: Simon and Schuster.

Dennison, P. 1985. *Personalized Whole-Brain Integration.* Ventura, Calif.: Educational Kinesiology Foundation. Available from the publisher. P. O. Box 3396, Ventura, CA 93006, (805) 650-3303.

———. 1986. *Brain Gym.* Ventura, Calif.: Educational Kinesiology Foundation. Available from the publisher. P. O. Box 3396, Ventura, CA 93006, (805) 650-3303.

———. 1994. *Brain Gym* Teacher's Edition, Revised. Ventura, Calif.: Educational Kinesiology Foundation. Available from the publisher. P. O. Box 3396, Ventura, CA 93006, (805) 650-3303.

Dobson, T. 1978. *Giving in to Get Your Way.* New York: Delacorte Press.

———. 1985. "A Kind Answer." In Heckler *Aikido and the New Warrior.*

Hannaford, C. 1993. *Education in Motion: A Practical Guide to Whole-Brain Body Integration for Everyone.* Video. Available from Zephyr Press.

———. 1995. *Smart Moves: Why Learning Is Not All in Your Head.* Arlington, Va.: Great Ocean Publishers. Available from the publisher. 1823 N. Lincoln St. Arlington, VA 22207-3746, (703) 525-0909.

Heckler, R. S., ed. 1985. *Aikido and the New Warrior.* Berkeley: New Atlantic Books.

Houston, J. 1980. *Lifeforce.* New York: Delacorte Press.

———. 1982. *The Possible Human.* Los Angeles: J.P. Tarcher. Includes the original forms of all of the exercises adapted in this book.

———. 1987. *Search for the Beloved.* Los Angeles: J.P. Tarcher.

Houston, J., and R. Masters. 1978. *Listening to the Body.* New York: Delacorte.

Leonard, G. 1974. *The Ultimate Athlete*. Berkeley: North Atlantic.
———. 1978. *The Silent Pulse*. New York: Dutton.
———. 1983. *Leonard Energy Training, A Trainer's Manual*. Mill Valley, Calif.: Energy Training Institute. Available from the publisher. P. O. Box 258, Mill Valley, CA, 94942.
———. 1992. *Mastery*. New York: Plume.
Leonard, G. and M. Murphy. 1995. *The Life We Are Given*. New York: Tarcher/Putnam.
Murphy, Michael. 1992. *The Future of the Body*. New York: Putnam/Karcher.
Patterson, M. and E. Wortz. 1976. *Magic Sam*. Bakersfield, Calif.: Patterson Learning Services. Available from the publisher. P. O. Box 2206, Bakersfield, CA 93303, (805) 833-0453.
Patterson, M. and E. Wortz. 1977. *Getting It Together with Rochester Rhinoceros*. Bakersfield, Calif.: Patterson Learning Services. Available from the publisher.
Rohnke, K. 1984. *Silver Bullets: A Guide of Initiative Problems, Adventure Games, and Trust Activities*. Dubuque, Iowa: Kendall/Hunt.

Organizations, Publishers, and Presenters

Multiple Intelligences

Zephyr Press. (Publisher, Presenter) Offers professional development conferences as well as an abundant range of books and teaching materials. P. O. Box 66006, Tucson, AZ 85728-6006, (520) 322-5090.

English and Second Languages

Berty Segal, Inc. (Presenter) Seminars and materials for using Total Physical Response (TPR). 1749 Eucalyptus, Brea, CA 92621, (714) 529-5379.

Richard Shope. (Presenter) Mime Media Instructional Technologies. *M.I.M.E. Writing Interactive Video Curriculum.* P. O. Box 4225, Whittier, CA 90607, (310) 693-9053.

Teachers' Discovery. (Publisher) Shakespeare rap tapes: *Romeo and Juliet* and *Julius Caesar*. P.O. Box 7048, Troy, MI 48007, (800) 543-4180.

Social Sciences

Teachers' Curriculum Institute. (Publisher, Presenter) *History Alive!* materials and seminars. 4149 El Camino Way, Ste B, Palo Alto, CA 94306-4010, (800) 497-6138.

Mathematics and Natural Sciences

Algebra Project, Inc. (Organization, Publisher) Effective, multimodal algebra teaching techniques. Highly successful with disadvantaged students grades 6–8. 99 Bishop Richard Allen Drive, Cambridge, MA, (617) 491-0200.

Lawrence Hall of Science University of California. (Publisher) Thematic teaching of science and mathematics. Berkeley, CA 94720, (510) 642-7771.

NASA/Jet Propulsion Laboratory, Pluto Educational Outreach. (Publisher, Organization) Richard Shope, Curriculum Development Lead. Curriculum guides and videotape available to schools at no cost. NASA/Jet Propulsion Laboratory, Mail Stop 301-250D, 4800 Oak Grove Drive, Pasadena, CA 91109, (818) 354-3812. E-mail address: pluto.education@jpl.nasa.gov.

Study Skills, Self-Management and Conflict Resolution

Educational Kinesiology Foundation. (Publisher, Organization) P.O. Box 3396, Ventura, CA 93006, (805) 650-3303.

George Leonard. (Presenter) Energy Training Institute, P. O. Box 258, Mill Valley, CA 94942.

All Core Subjects

Gail Herman. (Presenter) Seminars: *Moving Mnemonics, Kinesthetic Methods of Teaching and Learning.* 166 Lodge Circle, Swanton, MD 21561.

Interact. (Publisher) Outstanding simulation activities. Suggestion: When you use these activities, it's helpful to organize the teacher's guide and other items such as handouts in a three-ring binder. Many simulations include separate cards giving clues, challenges, or twists of fate. If you perforate envelopes to hold these cards, they can be kept handy in the three-ring binder along with your other materials. 1825 Gillespie Way 101, El Cajon, CA 92020, (619) 448-1474, (800) 359-0961.

Marilyn Nikimaa Patterson. (Presenter) *MI, Conflict Resolution,* and *Shakespeare for Kids.* P. O. Box 2206, Bakersfield, CA 93303, (805) 324-1891, (805) 833-0453.

Richard Shope. (Presenter) Seminar: *The Kinesthetic Connection across the Curriculum,* and Mime Media Instructional Technologies. Shope is also Curriculum Development Lead for the Pluto Educational Outreach Project at NASA/JPL (listed in the Math and Science section). P. O. Box 4225, Whittier, CA 90607, (800) 407-7959, (310) 693-9053.

Smithsonian Institution. (Publisher) *Resource Guide for Teachers* lists about 400 free and inexpensive items available from several museums and organizations: posters, slides, video and audiotapes, etc. Up to nine copies free. Office of Secondary and Elementary Education, Arts and Industries Building, Room 1163, MRC 402, Washington, D.C. 20560, (202) 357-2425.

Service Learning

National Youth Leadership Council. (Organization) 1910 W. County Rd. B, Roseville, MN 55113, (612) 631-3672, (800) 366-6952.

Youth Service America. (Organization) 1319 F Street, N.W., Washington, D.C. 20004, (202) 783-8855.